EAT FOR HEALTH

LOSE WEIGHT · KEEP IT OFF · LOOK YOUNGER · LIVE LONGER

Joel Fuhrman, M.D.

PUBLISHED BY

ዋ

Gift of Health Press

Original Edition, Published in a 2 book hardcover set
by Gift of Health Press, March 2008
Revised single paperback edition, September 2012

Contact:
Gift of Health Press
Flemington, NJ 08822
for wholesale inquires go to:
giftofhealthpress.com

Printed in the United States
ISBN: 9780983795223

Library of Congress Control Number:
2011941080

Publishers Note:
Keep in mind that results vary from person to person. Some people have a
medical history and/or condition that may warrant individual recommendations and in some cases drugs and even surgery. Do not start, stop or change
medication without professional medical advice, and do not change your diet
if you are ill or on medication except under the supervision of a competent
physician. Neither this, nor any other book, is intended to take the place of
personalized medical care or treatment.

ợp

Gift of Health Press

Book Design: Robyn Rolfes — Creative Syndicate, Inc.

TABLE OF CONTENTS

Prepare For A New You!

Congratulations on starting this program! Your decision to pursue superior health is one of the most important journeys you will ever undertake.

I developed *Eat for Health* after a comprehensive review of thousands of scientific studies on human nutrition conducted over the last 20 years. I can say with certainty that this is the place to begin your nutritional turnaround. I have seen the effects of this plan in action on thousands of patients with a wide range of diseases and health concerns, from migraines and allergies to heart disease and diabetes, and the bottom line is, it works. Superior nutrition is the foundation of this diet. It is the path to medical wellness in your own life. It is the most powerful intervention, not only to prevent disease, but also to reverse it. Complete recovery from most chronic degenerative illnesses is possible.

Nothing shows the power of this way of eating more than hearing from people who apply this knowledge and live it every day. Throughout this book, beginning with Chapter One's selection of medical case studies, you will find the testimonies of a sampling of people from around the country who have changed their lives following this plan. They are from different backgrounds, are different ages, and had different reasons for beginning this journey, but they all now share excellent health. As you make your way through this book, take a moment to think about their stories and to discover the advantages that are possible when you eat right and make a commitment to your own health.

The body is a self-healing machine when you supply it with an optimal nutritional environment. The information presented here is the fastest and most effective way to create that environment. If you have high blood pressure, high cholesterol, diabetes, heart disease, indigestion, headaches, asthma, fatigue, body aches, or pain—or you want to protect yourself from developing these and other chronic conditions—this plan is for you. *Eat for Health* can enable you to avoid angioplasty, bypass surgery, and other invasive procedures. By adopting this eating style early enough, you can make sure that you never have a heart attack, stroke, or dementia. You can reduce and eventually eliminate your need for prescription drugs. In short, you can not only optimize your health and potentially save your life, but do it all while increasing the pleasure you get from food.

Many of you are interested in this program because you want to lose weight. I want to assure you that you will lose all the weight you want, even if diets have failed you in the past, and the results will be permanent, not temporary. According to a recent medical study of over 760 participants, those adhering to my nutrient-rich diet-style lost addictive cravings and experienced a reduction in their desire to overeat.[1] This is not dieting; rather, it involves the biochemical repair of your appetite control. More and more, new medical studies are investigating and demonstrating that diets rich in high-nutrient plant foods have a suppressive effect on appetite and are the most effective for long-term weight control.[2] The healthiest way to eat is also the most successful way to obtain a favorable weight, if you consider long term results.

This is not a diet in the sense of something you do to lose weight.

This is a new diet-style for life. A diet-style that every American has the right to know about, so that they have the choice to protect their precious health. It is healthful eating. Eating healthfully is more effective for long-term weight control because it modifies and diminishes the sensations of so-called hunger, making it possible to be more comfortable eating fewer calories. I will talk about this later.

Many of my patients have lost up to 20 pounds in six weeks and that was just the beginning. However, this is nothing like your typical diet book because when the focus is on weight loss alone, the results are rarely permanent. Here, there is no calorie counting, portion-size measuring, or weighing involved. You will eat as much food as you want and over time you will become satisfied with fewer calories.

When you consume sufficient nutrients and fiber, you will become biochemically filled (nutrients) and mechanically filled (fiber), and your desire to consume calories will be blunted or turned down. One key factor that determines whether you will be overweight is your failure to consume sufficient fiber and nutrients.

This is an eating-style that you will learn to enjoy forever. You will be presented with logical, scientific information that explains the connection between diet and your health. Let these facts change the way you think about food. Incorporate the information into your life by using the *Eat for Health* meal plans and great tasting recipes. If you need to lose weight, you will shed pounds naturally and almost miraculously, merely as a side effect of eating so healthfully.

The reason my program works so well is because its success is built on knowledge. It takes time and effort to acquire this knowledge, but that's because this program is not simply a quick fix. Once you have learned and practiced all of the information, you will be a nutritional expert and the key to successful weight management will be in your hands—and your mind. This book will guide you through your transition as you step up to greater health. You will learn how to plan great menus and shop wisely for delicious, natural ingredients.

Applying the information in this book to your life will help you achieve long term success. It will create new, healthful behaviors that will eventually become effortless. It is so highly effective that it will enable you to take control of your own health destiny.

What Is *Eat to Live?*

Eat To Live is the title of my *New York Times* #1 best-selling book published in 2003 (revised and updated in 2011). People now use that phrase to describe my overwhelmingly successful eating-style. I happily receive a continuous barrage of e-mails and letters of gratitude describing miraculous changes in health which result from eating this way. Those testimonies—some of which you will read in these pages—encouraged me to develop *Eat for Health*.

Writing *Eat To Live* and seeing the miraculous changes it made in people's lives reinforced my belief that high-nutrient diets can restore the body to good health. Thousands of people lost dramatic amounts of weight without difficulty and never regained it back. More importantly, they recovered from diseases such as allergies, asthma, acne, headaches, high blood pressure, diabetes, reflux esophagitis, lupus, kidney insufficiency, angina, cardiomyopathy, multiple sclerosis, and many more. The results and success stories are astounding. I have long studied and utilized high-nutrient eating as a medical therapy, but even I have been surprised by the power of eating this way.

My intention in writing this book was to make the principles of *Eat To Live* easier to incorporate in your life. I also want to share new lessons I've learned about the obstacles people encounter when making dietary changes. This book makes the *Eat To Live* principles more accessible to a larger audience. You will see that all people—sick or healthy, overweight or slim, young or old—can benefit from this plan. It creates the environment necessary for our bodies to thrive and experience what amounts to a miracle in our modern world: a long, disease-free life without heart disease, strokes, dementia, or even cancer.

Even though the information presented here is an extension of the nutritional and lifestyle program I laid out in *Eat To Live*, you do not have to read *Eat To Live* to understand this program. When you encounter the words "*Eat To Live*," keep in mind that it simply refers to a way of eating, a combination of food and lifestyle factors that I have coined a word for, "nutritarian". Simply put, a nutritarian is a person who strives for more micronutrients per calorie in their diet-style. A nutritarian understands that food has powerful disease-protecting and therapeutic effects and seeks to consume a broad array of micronutrients via their food choices. This book will show you why it is important to become a nutritarian. Everything you need to achieve your health and weight-loss goals is in the pages before you. All you need to do is read them and incorporate the information into your daily life.

Nutrients: The Basis of the Program
The eating-style that you will find in these pages is based on a central idea: Most people do not consume enough micronutrients on a daily basis. Because their micronutrient needs aren't met, they can't control food cravings and overeating. This deficiency also makes them more susceptible to the critical diseases and serious medical conditions that plague the American population.

Micronutrients are vitamins, minerals, and phytochemicals: valuable, calorie-free parts of certain foods. My nutritional plan radically reduces your consumption of low-nutrient foods and radically increases your intake of high-nutrient foods. This program will never ask you to count calories, but for good health and a long, disease-free life we must seek to consume more nutrients from fewer calories. Basically, we must eat foods with a high nutritional bang per caloric buck.

Nutrient-density is the critical concept I use in giving dietary and nutritional advice to my patients and to the public. Adequate consumption of vitamins, minerals, and phytochemicals is essential for a healthy immune system and to empower your body's detoxification and cellular repair mechanisms to protect you from cancer and other diseases. In this book, I will show you how to choose foods that have the highest nutrient density and how to put together delicious menus that will allow you to reach new levels of superior nutrition.

Perhaps not surprisingly, you will find that most of the foods that have a high nutrient-density are straight from nature, primarily fruits and vegetables. These foods play major roles in the journey to great health. Nutritional science in the last 20 years has demonstrated that colorful plant foods contain a huge assortment of protective compounds, most of which are still being discovered and studied by scientists. We are learning that these compounds work in fascinating ways to detoxify carcinogens, repair DNA damage, reduce free radical formation and facilitate the removal of toxins from the body. Only by eating an assortment of nutrient rich natural foods can we obtain the diversity of elements needed to protect ourselves from common diseases.

You Are the Cure

I have been part of the medical community as a family physician for more than 20 years, and I can tell you that drugs and doctors cannot grant you excellent health and protection from disease and suffering. Almost every doctor knows this. The most effective health-care is self-care. Reading this book, practicing the plan and mastering its techniques will provide the best possible self-care: superior nutrition. The superior nutrition I'm describing can prevent and even reverse most medical problems within three to six months. This is a bold claim, but the facts, supported by scientific research and literature, show that most medical problems and medical tragedies we face in the modern world are the result of nutritional folly. Our American diet has resulted in a sickly nation with the majority of people taking prescription drugs by the time they reach the age of 50. Your body is made of the foods you have eaten, and when you eat the standard American diet (SAD), you get the diseases that most other Americans get.

Forty percent of Americans die of heart attacks and strokes. You don't have to be one of them. Twenty-eight million Americans suffer from the crippling pain of osteoarthritis. You don't have to be one of them. Thirty-five million Americans suffer from chronic headaches. You don't have to be one of them. You simply do not have to be sick.

We consider it normal to lose youthful vigor in our thirties, carry 30 to 40 extra pounds, live with chronic illness in our late forties and fifties, only to live our last decades completely dependent on others. This should not be considered normal. This is the result of a life-long pattern of unhealthful living and misguided information. We should look forward to enjoying an active life into our nineties. This seems like an outrageous expectation because most people spend a lifetime consuming an inadequate diet. They have yet to make the connection that we are what we eat and that ill health in the later years of our lives is the result of our earlier, poor choices.

Most of the thousands of patients I have treated first came to my office unhappy, sick, and overweight, having tried every dietary craze without success. Many, following this educational program for superior health and weight loss, shed the weight they always dreamed of losing and kept it off. For the first time in their lives they had a diet plan that didn't require them to be hungry all the time. Most importantly, they were able to eventually discontinue their medications. When you learn and follow this program of eating it is possible to:

- Never have a heart attack or a stroke

- Avoid dementia in later life

- Dramatically reduce your chance of getting cancer

- Prevent and heal digestive problems such as reflux, dyspepsia, constipation, and hemorrhoids

- Prevent and often resolve erectile impotence, high blood pressure, and other circulatory impairments

- Prevent and reverse diabetes (Type II) and high cholesterol, at first lessening the need for drugs and eventually resolving these conditions

- Age slower, live longer, and maintain youthful vigor, intelligence, and productivity into the later years

Some people may be skeptical that I can make such radical claims, but these statements are supported by medical science and thousands of clinical patient case histories. The reversal of dietary-caused diseases occurs in a relatively short time and is easily achieved by anyone following my program.

Be One of the Few, Not the Many
Like the classic victim, we actually grow to love those things that are killing us—in this case, food. This phenomenon is known as addiction and an addiction to certain foods can be just as deadly as many other addictions. However, if you are reading this, it is not too late to change. I can show you how to get rid of the food addictions sabotaging your health.

Since you have purchased this book, you are probably interested in the relationship between what you eat and your health. It is likely you are already attempting to eat differently than those around you. The secret to achieving spectacular results is your willingness to become informed and knowledgeable about modern nutritional science and not be held back by prior misinformed beliefs. I offer you this simple idea: if you adopt this program, you will achieve your ideal weight, slow down the clock of aging, and prevent and even reverse disease, all at the same time. While doing this, you will also discover a level of enjoyment with eating that you have never imagined. It all begins with a state of mind, but you first must be open to the possibility that this can happen.

Your success is dependent on your willingness to learn. It is okay if you don't want to adopt everything in this program or even agree with everything you read at first. The way to get the most out of this book is to read it completely. I recommend you suspend decision making at first. It is best if you wait until you have learned more, then you will be in an educated position to decide if you really do disagree with something and why. Try not to let what you have learned in the past cloud your learning here; nutritional science has changed dramatically in recent years. This scientific, nutritional program was designed after years of studying thousands of articles from the scientific literature, seeing the most effective nutritional interventions used by other physicians around the world, and observing and testing these methods with my patients. The preponderance of evidence points in the same direction: the program works and it works best for those who understand it best. Read, practice the exercises, and ask questions. Those who learn and understand this program typically find they achieve remarkable results.

What is *Eat for Health*?

Eat for Health is designed to make this eating-style easy and fun by combining my nutritional knowledge and experience with motivational exercises, new cooking techniques, sample menus and delicious recipes. I have developed and used this information with thousands of patients over the years with remarkable results.

The first chapters of this book cover the fundamentals of superior nutrition; you will learn to overcome the obstacles that are preventing you from adopting a healthy eating-style for life. You will start to get ready for your new eating-style by doing my Exercises with Food. As you complete your *Eat for Health* journey, you will learn about three different levels/phases of nutrient-density. Each level incorporates more nutritional principles to disease-proof your body. Level 3 is the most effective eating-style for reversing disease and maximizing health and longevity. If you are struggling with an autoimmune disease, cancer or other serious illness, you will want to target Level 3 as your optimal diet. Otherwise, I find that Level 2 provides an excellent level of nutrient density for most of my patients. Any of the levels will bring you closer to your health goals and if you are overweight, you will see dramatic benefits with all levels.

I have designed weekly menu plans with recipes for each level. You can pick a level and stay with it or start at Level 1 and gradually progress to Level 2 or 3. The menu plans also allow you the option of moving back and forth between levels by making small but significant additions to your diet. As you learn more and work with this book, your taste buds will gradually realign themselves and actually become stronger and more discriminating. As you become healthier, you will lose your psychological dependence on empty-calorie foods. One of the ways in which *Eat for Health* is unique and revolutionary is that it is based on the idea of gradual implementation of an increasingly higher micronutrient content in a person's diet. Where many diets ask you to go cold turkey on certain foods, or make the first weeks of their plans the hardest, this program is designed so you can make smaller changes first. As you increase your knowledge and preference for healthy foods, you can choose to move forward—all at your own pace.

As you increase your intake of nutrient dense foods and replace unhealthful foods, you will, over a period of time, reset your internal taste preferences and hunger drive. Once this happens, you will be amazed at how easy it becomes to follow my plan and maintain your ideal weight forever, without dieting.

Using This Book

Go at your own pace. I advise you to master the material and exercises in each chapter before moving on to the next one. The goal of this program is to teach you to eat healthfully, enjoy it, and learn to prefer a nutritarian eating-style instead of a disease-promoting one. Don't decide now whether you think you can do it or whether you want to make all these changes. Learn the material before making a judgment; give the information a chance to work. It may be that the change from the way you eat now to Level 1 of this eating-style is a big one. If so, you can make this first big change and stop there for a while. It's all up to you.

To help you see your progress, I have given foods ANDI or nutrient density scores. These numbers are a way to quantify the nutritional content of a variety of different foods and will help you learn which foods you should be choosing on a daily basis.

This Is a Different Diet World

I know how frustrating it is to dive into a promising diet only to meet with failure. You blame yourself, which sets up a vicious cycle of guilt and punishment. This expresses itself through self-defeating behavior. Most people who have been through this cycle have given up on the idea of reaching their ideal weight. It seems impossible and their failure in the past reinforces this. That will not be the case here. Mediocre expectations yield mediocre results, so you must, right now, raise your expectations. Give this program a true test and follow it as directed, and I am confident you will get different results than you have in the past. You will not only lose your excess weight, but you will also see both subtle and dramatic improvements in your health. You will lower your cholesterol, triglycerides, and blood pressure. If you have adult-onset (Type II) diabetes, it will improve and can eventually resolve. Most people are amazed as symptoms such as migraines, acid reflux, and indigestion disappear. You will experience the power of health.

I feel strongly that this is the most effective diet for disease-protection and longevity, and, if you are significantly overweight, it is also the most safe and effective way to lose a dramatic amount of weight. It works for those who have failed at losing weight or achieving their dietary goals in the past. Studies have shown that only three out of 100 people who attempt to lose weight actually succeed. The problem is not people. The problem is that most weight-loss approaches focus on reducing calories, which winds up reducing nutrients simultaneously, and is predictive of eventual failure.

The cuisine designed for superior nutrition is radically different from other plans because you eat a lot of food. Forget calorie counting and traditional diets. Don't panic because you feel full and satisfied; this is normal. If you are overweight, you will still lose weight. Your body appreciates the nutrients and will reward you with optimal health and an ideal weight.

CAUTION:

This program is so effective at dropping your weight, blood pressure, and blood sugar that medication adjustments will be necessary so that you are not over-medicated. If your blood sugar or blood pressure improves dramatically and medications are not reduced or eliminated, it could be harmful to your health. Please consult your physician.

Finding Your Motivation

You are what you eat. To be your best, you must eat the best. Perhaps you already know this, but it doesn't always make it easy to live that way. I will teach you new nutritional principles which will enable you to change the way you think and improve your health. I can also teach you to prefer to eat healthfully if you give me that chance, but motivation is key to starting the program and sticking with it.

On a scale of 1 to 10, rate the most compelling reasons you have for eating healthfully:

_____ I want to recover from a chronic illness, such as high blood pressure, diabetes, headaches, or high cholesterol.

_____ I want to protect myself from developing a dangerous disease.

_____ I want to prevent the deterioration in health, physical, and mental abilities that are typically considered a normal part of aging.

_____ I want to lose weight and look and feel better.

_____ I want to increase my energy and reduce fatigue.

_____ I want to improve the health of my family.

_____ I want to improve my physical fitness.

_____ I want protection from frequent bouts of infectious disease.

_____ I want to have better digestion.

_____ I want to have better sexual enjoyment and performance.

_____ I want to look and feel younger.

_____ I want to have a better emotional outlook on life.

_____ I want to live longer.

_____ I want to live without medical interference and hospitalizations.

_____ I want to avoid surgery or prescription medication.

_____ I want to reduce my dependency on medication.

_____ I want to save money on health care and prescription drugs.

Each time you feel some difficulty with the eating-style in this book, each time you want to revert back to your old ways of eating, each time you slip-up on the program, each time you believe this level of health is unattainable for you, come back and look at this page. Habits are hard to break and the way you eat is a habit. Remind yourself of how important these things are and why they are more than adequate motivation for continuing to learn, practice, and live with the goal of superior nutrition.

CHAPTER ONE

THOUSANDS OF SUCCESS STORIES

The nutritarian diet-style is the only way of eating that will allow you to shed pounds while you reverse existing diseases and protect yourself from future health problems. In the following pages, you will learn about the science that makes this way of eating successful in optimizing your health, and you will discover how to live this diet in your own life. However, what I often find even more convincing than the scientific data is seeing the results from patients who have followed my plan. For over 20 years, I have been recommending the fundamentals of this diet to the patients in my medical practice, the readers of my previous books, and people who have reached out to me from around the world. In that time, I have seen the transformative power of practicing an eating-style focused on high-nutrient foods, the core of this plan. Hearing from people who have lived this plan and seen these changes in their own lives is thrilling.

Below is a small sampling of the thousands of emails and letters that I have received from my patients and from people who have followed my nutritional advice and discovered the transformative power of this way of eating. The illnesses and weight problems detailed below vary greatly, but all of these individuals found that the power of prescription medicine was nothing compared to the power of nutrition. Browse through their stories, told in their own words, and let their personal experiences inform and motivate you in your quest for great health. You will understand better what the *Eat for Health* plan can do for you, and you will be ready to implement it in your life.

Cardiovascular Issues

"Five years ago, at the age of 49, my husband Don appeared to be in perfect health, but then he began to experience pressure in his chest. We found out that his left anterior descending artery was 95 percent blocked and his cholesterol was 259 with an LDL cholesterol of 178. He had a stent placed, remained under the care of cardiologists, and was taking cholesterol lowering drugs, high blood pressure medications, and blood thinners. He tried to eat more carefully too, but he began having chest discomfort again and was found to have further heart disease.

This time, while waiting to have more invasive procedures performed, a friend of ours who is a doctor told us about the work Dr. Fuhrman was doing and encouraged us to see him as quickly as possible.

When we first met him, we were so impressed with the time Dr. Fuhrman spent with us, reviewing Don's history and sharing a wealth of information in a way that we could understand. We returned home with all the tools we needed to get us started on the journey to regaining health. We thoroughly enjoyed *Eat To Live* and immediately began to implement the program. We were amazed at the results.

Within two weeks Don had lost twelve pounds and his blood pressure dropped so low he no longer needed medications. Now he is 20 pounds lighter, his chest pains are resolved, and he was able to discontinue all his medications. His LDL cholesterol went from 163 while he was on medication to 103 off medication— and I lost 10 pounds as well! We both want to thank Dr. Fuhrman for helping us understand how important it is to *'Eat To Live'* by giving our bodies the food we need for proper nutrition. We just can't thank him enough for everything."

Laura and Don Klase
Orefield, Pennsylvania

LUPUS

"When I was 32 years old, I developed a rash on my face, and my body felt stiff and sore. The joint pain in my hands and shoulders continued to worsen, and my wrists felt like someone had hit them with a hammer. I saw a rheumatologist who prescribed an anti-inflammatory drug and blood work. It indicated that I had lupus. At first I thought, 'Good news. I have a diagnosis, so now I can do something about it.' I became discouraged when I was told there is no known cure for lupus. I would have to live with the disease and be on medication, including steroids, for the rest of my life. I was also told that I could experience serious organ damage, need a kidney transplant, and die. In addition, the medicine would make me gain weight and be puffy.

This information was not acceptable to me. I searched for answers, and, after trying other things with no success, I found Dr. Fuhrman. I traveled from Virginia to his office in New Jersey. I followed his advice regarding eating a high-nutrient diet, and, within a few months, I had made a complete recovery from lupus. For the first time in years, I looked and felt great. I visited my old rheumatologist because I thought he would be impressed with my story.

When I told him about my experience and my newfound health he wrote 'Spontaneous Recovery' on my chart and dismissed me rudely. So, when a doctor tells you that it has not been proven that diet has any effect on lupus, keep in mind that he may never have listened to people who told him otherwise. Today, lupus is not part of my life. I play tennis and compete on a local team, and no one would guess that I was ever in so much pain."

Robin Zelman
Charlottesville, Virginia

ASTHMA, MIGRAINES AND HIGH BLOOD PRESSURE

"By the age of 43, I was a physical mess. I was 70 pounds overweight, asthma had become a constant nuisance in my life, and I had developed high blood pressure, acid reflux, and an irregular heartbeat. I was especially concerned because heart problems cost both my parents their lives at young ages. I was on blood pressure medications, four Tums, and two different inhalers. I also frequently required oral steroids. I was sent to a dietician who told me I would lose 10 pounds if I changed from drinking Coke to Diet Coke. For years I saw an allergist once a week for allergy shots. Then I started to experience violent migraines on a frequent basis, which was the last straw. One day a friend gave me a newspaper article about Dr. Fuhrman's work and I called his office immediately.

Dr. Fuhrman's advice totally transformed my life and the lives of many of my friends. Six years later, I no longer have headaches. I have not needed asthma medications in years and I do not have high blood pressure anymore. I have lost 70 pounds and kept it off. I thank God for my good health and the high energy level I experience every-day. I realize that all my years of medical problems were self-caused by my food choices. Now my husband and I enjoy each meal from a repertoire of delicious, healthy recipes, and I can't imagine living any other way."

Linda Castagna
Milford, New Jersey

SARCOIDOSIS

"I was generally thin until I turned 32; then I gained 30 pounds almost overnight. At age 34, I began having labored breathing and was diagnosed with sarcoidosis. The disease caused significant scarring over a large area of my lungs. I began the standard treatment of a biopsy and steroids.

Another three years and 20 pounds later, my life changed when the button on my last comfortable pair of pants snapped and the zipper broke. It was funny and embarrassing, but deadly serious all at the same time. That day I decided I had to change and went to the bookstore to find some answers. I stumbled upon Dr. Fuhrman's book, and it made sense to me.

Six months later, I was 60 pounds lighter. Then my wife noticed a lump on my neck. It had been there for years, but without all my fat obscuring it, it was now readily visible. I had assumed that my gasping was the result of the sarcoidosis, but it turned out I had a massive thyroid cyst blocking my windpipe and cutting off my air supply. The doctors decided that it needed to come out.

Prior to surgery, I had an MRI and the doctors found I had no traces of sarcoidosis. It had completely cleared up, just as Dr. Fuhrman had predicted. The surgery was problematic and I went into anaphylactic shock because the walls of my thyroid were stretched to the limit.

I almost died, but more sobering was the fact that if I hadn't followed Dr. Fuhrman's advice, the cyst would have remained obscured and burst on its own.

I am now 46 years old; I run 20 miles each week and have unbelievable stamina. My systolic blood pressure went from 140 to 108, and my current LDL cholesterol level is 40. I feel great, look 10 years younger than I did two years ago, and take no medications. You too can achieve your ideal weight, reverse disease, and delay the aging process!"

Bob Phillips
Morrestown, New Jersey

Psoriasis And Psoriatic Arthritis

"I was desperate when I traveled to New Jersey to see Dr. Fuhrman. I had been diagnosed with psoriatic arthritis and had suffered from open skin lesions and full body itchiness for years. I followed his advice to the letter. He put me on a special eating plan, and, after about three months, I started to get better. My legs and arms cleared up first. My body healed from the extremities inward, and six months later my psoriasis was totally gone. My doctors are amazed. Today my skin is completely clear with no itchiness or blotches, and I have no more arthritic pain. Recent blood tests show I no longer have the blood test markers that show inflammation. I cannot fully express what this recovery means to me. I am so grateful that Dr. Fuhrman insisted I could be helped and then guided me to wellness."

Jodi O'Neil
Cary, North Carolina

POLYMYALGIA AND FIBROMYALGIA

"I developed joint pains when I was 40 years old and then found out I had high blood pressure and high cholesterol. I went on the Atkins diet and my cholesterol shot up to over 300. My body aches and pains worsened and I was diagnosed with polymyalgia rheumatica and then fibromyalgia, a condition of chronic pain. I couldn't sleep well. I couldn't even sit on the toilet without severe pain. I took medications, steroids, and even used magnets, but nothing helped. I prayed and got to the point where I didn't even want to live if my life had to be like this.

Then a co-worker told me about the best health book she had ever read. It was *Eat to Live*. I read it in two days, and I still read it over and over again like a textbook. It has been two years since I first got the book and today I am well. I can even work out at the gym four times a week. Many people think that eating unhealthy food is the most important thing, but I have learned that feeling great is even more important. I am 66 and I feel better than I did when I was 30."

Suzanne Demeo
South Orange, New Jersey

DIABETES AND DIABETIC RETINOPATHY

"Before I read Dr. Fuhrman's book I weighed 205 pounds and had diabetes for seven years. The information enabled me to lose 60 pounds and get rid of my diabetes, high blood pressure, and high cholesterol without medication. My LDL cholesterol went from 168 to 73 in five months, and I successfully dropped my weight to 143 pounds. The most amazing thing is that my ophthalmologist had told me that I required laser surgery to treat diabetic retinopathy, but after changing my diet he found that the damage was no longer there and I didn't require surgery. I am extremely grateful because I know Dr. Fuhrman has added many quality years to my life."

Martin Milford
Santa Rosa, California

SEVERE MIGRAINES AND FATIGUE

"Our daughter Renee has been plagued by headaches since she was five. They intensified when she was 11 and from that point on she suffered tremendously from the pain and the treatments she had to endure. In addition to an arsenal of drugs, she was hospitalized four times and even received intravenous drugs; nothing worked We went to chiropractors, nutritionists, dentists, acupuncturists, and rheumatologists, but nothing helped. Renee was not able to remain in school. She was tutored at home when she felt up to it, but most of the time she simply could not get out of bed.

As you can imagine, this had a profound impact on Renee and our family. She was forced to give up sports, trips, friends, school, and just being a kid. Twice she talked about not wanting to live anymore. As a result, she began seeing a counselor to help her deal with this life-altering illness.

I did not consider Renee an unhealthy eater, but at her first visit to Dr. Fuhrman he tested her level of antioxidants and carotenoids and found them to be extremely low. He explained that Renee's deficiencies of these nutrients were preventing her body from effectively removing metabolic wastes and other toxins. He told us it would take about three months for her to get well. We were highly skeptical, but Renee gave it her best shot. Our entire family ate Dr. Fuhrman's vegetable-based diet and truly enjoyed the recipes.

After one month I was still concerned because Renee did not seem better and was still suffering. I called Dr. Fuhrman and he reminded me that getting the nutrients into Renee's bloodstream did not mean those nutrients were concentrated in her skin, brain, and other tissues.

After three months, Renee was her old self again. She was smiling all the time and her headaches were almost totally gone. Her energy and personality returned, she has resumed school, and she's back doing sports again. I cried with joy when I saw Dr. Fuhrman again. He has given us our daughter back."

Janine Kranor
Oakland, New Jersey

ULCERS

"For approximately a year before consulting with Dr. Fuhrman, our daughter Caitlin suffered from progressive fatigue, severe acne, and chronic stomach upset. It caused numerous absences from school, which was troubling because Caitlin was an honor student who had always done well academically. After seeing several doctors with no diagnosis, Caitlin became exceedingly frustrated and asked us to enroll her in counseling for stress management. We began counseling as a family.

Caitlin's symptoms worsened and she was eventually diagnosed with ulcers. Six weeks later, we learned that the tests revealed an alarmingly high presence of the antibodies that fight bacterially based ulcers. According to the doctor, Caitlin probably had the bacteria in her stomach for more than a year. He immediately prescribed a course of four antibiotics taken simultaneously, which destroyed her digestive system. She was worse than ever.

We asked our counselor to recommend a physician who practiced nutritional medicine and we were led to Dr. Fuhrman. He immediately put Caitlin on a cleansing diet with lots of green vegetables and high-nutrient soups, but no medication of any kind. Over those first two months, as her digestive system healed, Caitlin regained her energy and her skin cleared. No more stomach upset, no more acne, no more fatigue. Caitlin was healthy in body and spirit and she was discharged from counseling. She graduated from high school with honors and received a scholarship to pursue her college education. We are so grateful to Dr. Fuhrman and nutritional medicine and can't imagine where we would be without this approach."

Gigi Smith
West Milford, New Jersey

Fertility

"My husband is a physician, and when he and I first found out about Dr. Fuhrman, we were both very impressed with his depth of knowledge. We converted to the plant-based approach to eating, and we increased our energy levels, lowered our cholesterol, and lost excess weight. Surprisingly, we were then able to conceive our first child. Subsequently, I enjoyed two complication-free pregnancies, which is no small detail since I gave birth at age 39 and 44. That was not a possibility before I started following Dr. Fuhrman's nutritional recommendations.

Our nutrition choices have continued to change our lives and the lives of our children. Because they have always eaten a high nutrient, plant-based diet, they enjoy fruits and vegetables, and mealtime is a pleasant experience. Neither of them has ever needed antibiotics. They have had no ear infections, allergies, asthma, or persistent childhood illnesses."

Sheila Ott
Greensboro, North Carolina

DEPRESSION

"I suffered for many years going from doctor to doctor, including alternative medicine doctors, and for the most part I got worse. I had severe migraines, depression, and anxiety, and was taking anti-depressants and pain-killers. I was gaining weight, becoming lethargic, and had just about given up. Then I started Dr. Fuhrman's plan. Within a few weeks, I was off all medications and losing weight. Amazingly, my headaches disappeared! However, years later I moved away from Dr. Fuhrman, I went through a stressful period and started eating how I used to. I became depressed, anxious and the headaches returned. I went to another doctor who insisted I go back on medication. One day, I was lying in a dark room, coping with a headache and I realized what I needed to do. I pulled out my books, re-started the program, and I am once again free of pain. I learned my lesson: you are what you eat."

Patti Brandt
Tucson, Arizona

"During spring and summer I was practically the girl in the bubble. My entire life revolved around avoiding exposure to things that would trigger my severe allergies and asthma. I never went outdoors, except long enough to get into my air-conditioned car that was equipped with a pollen filter. Then I started Dr. Fuhrman's plan and my symptoms got less and less severe. I used to associate nice weather with misery and my dangerous medications, but now it's smooth sailing! I feel so free! I can sit next to open windows and have no symptoms and even spend entire days outside. It's amazing: my allergies and asthma are gone!"

Jennifer McCay
Jersey City, New Jersey

The Facts and Figures

These limited case studies are only a tiny sampling of the many thousands of lives that have been dramatically changed for the better by adopting this program of high-nutrient eating. For example, so many of my patients have achieved recoveries from lupus that one of them interviewed other patients who had previously suffered from autoimmune diseases and wrote a book about it. Some physicians or skeptics may say, "You claim to have hundreds of documented cases of disease recoveries, but these case histories are not sufficient. You also need medical studies that can corroborate these results. Lots of people can make false claims. How do I know your word is true?"

My response is that I agree that more scientific studies would be helpful, and my office is involved with several new research trials. However, some very important research supporting these concepts has been done already, so these cases are not the only evidence that diseases such as high blood pressure, heart and circulatory diseases, diabetes, headaches, and digestive problems can be prevented and resolved via better nutrition. Before getting into the foundation of this program, let's briefly review a small sampling of the scientific evidence that supports this plan and helps explain the science behind the many health transformations that have occurred in people's lives.

As you move forward, keep in mind that there are other diets with some features of *Eat for Health*. Obviously, the scientific evidence over the last 50 years has encouraged many knowledge-able individuals to eat more plant-based foods. However, the small nuances that make this program unique make a big difference in the outcome, especially in achieving permanent results. Remember, temporary weight loss is of no benefit. The results must stick forever. *Eat for Health* gets the best results because it has no equal when motivating people to change for the long-term.

One of the features that makes this program work is learning about the healing power of high-nutrient super foods; however, that alone is not unique. *Eat for Health* explains and targets the most critical facets of what makes a diet medicinal. It supplies optimal levels of nutrients, while minimizing excesses and harm-ful food choices, and does it in a way that makes eating health-fully more pleasurable. It also prevents overeating and removes cravings and food addiction. To truly understand it, you must dive into this book.

Eat For Health and Cardiovascular Disease

The dietary recommendations contained in this book and the elements that make a diet cardio-protective have been tested in multiple studies. The evidence here is overwhelming. Let's first look at the LDL cholesterol lowering effects of various dietary plans, as documented in published medical journal articles.

METHOD	% DECREASE LDL CHOLESTEROL
American Heart Association standard low-fat advice[3]	6%
High protein (Atkins-type)[4]	No significant change
Low-fat vegetarian[5]	16%
High olive oil—Mediterranean[6]	No significant change
Cholesterol-lowering medication (statins)[7]	26%
Nutritarian (high-nutrient density)[8]	33%

Eating a nutritarian diet-style puts together many different qualities that make it cardioprotective and cholesterol-reducing. It's not just a low-fat or vegetarian way of eating that makes a diet ideal. This eating-style has such dramatic benefits because it is very high in mixed fibers and vegetables and has sterols and other compounds from beans and nuts. This is the only dietary intervention shown to lower cholesterol as effectively as cholesterol-lowering medications. Though the low-fat vegetarian diet did lower LDL cholesterol 16 percent, triglycerides were actually 18.7 percent higher and the LDL/HDL ratio remained unchanged. The results of the study that patterned the recommendations of *Eat for Health* differed in that the LDL cholesterol was more significantly lowered without unfavorable impact on HDL or triglycerides, reflecting sizable improvement in cardiac risk factors. I have hundreds of patients in my medical practice who have witnessed dramatic reductions in their blood lipids, especially LDL cholesterol, without drugs.

Keep in mind that cholesterol lowering does not adequately explain the protective effects of a nutritarian diet for cardiovascular disease since the diet has powerful anti-inflammatory and other beneficial biochemical effects. Even though drugs may lower cholesterol, they cannot be expected to offer the dramatic protection against cardiovascular events that superior nutrition can. The aggressive use of cholesterol-lowering drugs does not prevent most heart attacks and strokes and does not decrease the risk of fatal strokes.[9] That is, in clinical trials a significant percentage of patients on the best possible statin therapy still experience events; however, lowering cholesterol with superior nutrition can be expected to offer dramatically more protection and disease reversal compared to drug therapy, without the risk or expense of prescription medication. Consider these articles from the medical community:

1) The effect of a plant-based diet on plasma lipids in hypercholesterolemic adults: a randomized trial. *Annals of Internal Medicine* (2005)

   This study showed that when two diets have the same amount of fat and saturated fat, it is the one with the higher amount of high-nutrient plant material that gives the best results for cholesterol-lowering and other measurable disease risks. Here is the conclusion without modification:

   "Previous national dietary guidelines primarily emphasized avoiding saturated fat and cholesterol; as a result, the guidelines probably underestimated the potential LDL cholesterol-lowering effect of diet. In this study, emphasis on including nutrient-dense plant-based foods, consistent with recently revised national guidelines, increased the total and LDL cholesterol-lowering effect of a low-fat diet."[10]

2) The combination of high fruit and vegetable consumption with low saturated fat intake is more protective against mortality in aging men than is either alone: the Baltimore Longitudinal Study of Aging. *The Journal of Nutrition* (2005)

   This study showed that reducing saturated fat intake is helpful in reducing heart disease deaths, but in terms of the potential to reduce death from all causes it is not as effective as diets that are high in fresh vegetables and fruits. The study showed, however, that when there is a low saturated fat intake and a higher intake of vegetables, fruits and beans, the benefits are dramatic. Over an 18 year follow-up of more than 501 initially healthy men, these researchers found that when both parameters were met, men consuming more than five servings of fruits and vegetables per day and getting less than 12 percent of calories from saturated fat were 76 percent less likely to die of heart disease and 31 percent less likely to die from all-cause mortality (meaning all causes of death).

The study stated:

"These findings demonstrate that the combination of both behaviors is more protective than either alone, suggesting that their beneficial effects are mediated by different mechanisms." [11]

3) Plant-based foods and prevention of cardiovascular disease: an overview. *American Journal of Clinical Nutrition* (2003)

The study concluded:

"Evidence from prospective cohort studies indicates that a high consumption of plant-based foods such as fruit and vegetables, nuts, and whole grains is associated with a significantly lower risk of coronary artery disease and stroke. The protective effects of these foods are probably mediated through multiple beneficial nutrients contained in these foods, including antioxidant vitamins, minerals, phytochemicals, fiber, and plant proteins. In dietary practice, healthy plant-based diets do not necessarily have to be low in fat. Instead, these diets should include unsaturated fats as the predominant form of dietary fat such as nuts. Such diets, which also have many other health benefits, deserve more emphasis in dietary recommendations to prevent chronic diseases." [12]

These studies are representative of thousands that illustrate that superior nutrition could have profound effects on each of us and on the collective health of our nation. In my many years of medical practice caring for thousands of patients with advanced and even unstable heart disease, every one of the patients who adopted my nutritional advice for the long-term improved their cardiac condition, and not one that I'm aware of has experienced another heart attack. Many physicians using aggressive nutritional interventions for patients with heart disease, including Dean Ornish, M.D., have documented similar results.[13]

The evidence conclusively shows that the national dietary guidelines, and even the improved recommendations of the American Heart Association, do not go far enough to offer people the information necessary for maximizing results. Modern cardiology is focused on drugs and high-tech interventions that do little to extend lifespan. However, for those desiring more than mediocrity and a true protection against heart disease and premature death, there is a clear-cut answer. The most effective and safest way to lower your LDL cholesterol and protect your long-term health is through this health-altering and life-saving approach. The life that is saved could be yours.

Eat for Health and Diabetes

As the number of people with Type II (adult onset) diabetes continues to soar, it is openly recognized that the growing waistline of the modern world is the main cause of this epidemic. Most physicians, dietitians, and even the American Diabetes Association have virtually given up on weight reduction as the primary treatment for diabetics. Consider this statement from a medical advisory committee: "It is nearly impossible to take very obese people and get them to lose significant weight. So rather than specifying an amount of weight loss, we are targeting getting metabolic control." This is doublespeak for—our recommended diets don't work, so we just give medications and watch patients gradually deteriorate as the diabetes advances. Today, medications are the mainstay of treatment and, unfortunately, most of these medications cause weight gain, worsening the syndrome and making the individual more diabetic.

Additionally, the narrow focus on blood-sugar reduction and reliance on medications gives patients a false sense of security because they mistakenly think their somewhat better controlled glucose levels are an indication of restored or improved health. They continue to gain weight following the same dietary habits that originally caused the problem.

It is well accepted that if it were possible for people to stick with weight reduction and high-nutrient eating, that route would be the most successful. Patients with diabetes who successfully lose weight from undergoing gastric bypass surgery typically see their diabetes melt away.[14] Dietary programs that have been successful at affecting weight loss have been dramatically effective for diabetics too, enabling patients to discontinue medications.[15]

Preventing and reversing diabetes is not all about weight loss. The nutritional features of *Eat for Health* have profound effects on improving pancreatic function and lowering insulin resistance over and above what could be accomplished with weight loss alone. The increased fiber, micronutrients, and stool bulk, plus the cholesterol-lowering and anti-inflammatory effects of this eating-style, have dramatic effects on Type II diabetes. Scores of my patients have been able to restore their glucose levels to the normal range without any further need for medications. They have become non-diabetic. Even my thin, Type I, insulin-dependent diabetic patients are typically able to reduce their insulin requirements by almost half and have better glucose control using this high-nutrient eating-style.

Diets high in fiber and vegetables have been consistently shown to be beneficial for diabetic patients and offer considerably better results when compared to the current recommendations of the American Diabetic Association Diet.[16] The dietary advice typically offered to diabetics is not science-based, and it caters to Americans' food preferences and food addictions. In contrast, the qualities of this eating-style provide maximum benefits for weight reduction, cardio-protection, and diabetes reversal. My latest book, *The End of Diabetes* gives my total program for both Type 1 and Type 2 Diabetes.

Eat for Health and Autoimmune Disease

Working with patients who have autoimmune diseases is one of the most rewarding aspects of my medical practice. Autoimmune and immune-mediated illnesses include diseases such as rheumatoid arthritis, lupus, psoriasis, multiple sclerosis, connective tissue disease, and the inflammatory bowel diseases called ulcerative colitis and Crohn's, but there are also more than 100 clinical syndromes considered autoimmune diseases.

This book describes the critical features of the eating style most effective in reversing or controlling these conditions. Obviously, not every patient with these diseases can make a complete, drug-free recovery; however, the amazing thing is that so many patients can, and do, recover. The recoveries are not limited to recognized autoimmune diseases. I see many patients with pain syndromes without laboratory documentation of autoimmune disease. The ability to achieve substantial improvement, and in many cases complete remission of these supposedly incurable illnesses, is exciting. I have been writing about these success stories for many years, including submissions to medical publications.[17] For the last 20 years, multiple studies have been published in medical journals documenting the effectiveness of high-vegetable diets on autoimmune illnesses.[18] These have been largely ignored by the medical profession and most doctors still deny the effectiveness of nutrition on autoimmune and inflammatory conditions. Although it is not clear why these studies are quickly forgotten or ignored after their publication, one factor may be that there is no financial incentive for anyone to promote the power of dietary intervention as a medical therapy. Pharmaceutical companies however, make large profits when studies show some efficacy for their products.

CHAPTER TWO

DISCOVERING NEW HEALTH

"I first came to see Dr. Fuhrman because I had high blood pressure and high cholesterol. Even given my medical conditions, I didn't want to give up many of my favorite foods. I was shocked when he told me, 'Then don't.' Instead, he asked me to add food to my diet by eating more vegetables. After the first week, I couldn't believe it: I actually liked eating raw vegetables and making great salad dressings. I added a pound of raw vegetables to my diet each day and lost ten pounds that month—without going on a diet at all! Of course, Dr. Fuhrman was right; I simply did not need to eat so much of the foods I thought I could not live without. After three months, he tricked me. Without making me give up any of my 'favorites,' I chose on my own to eat very little of them. Now, I've lost over 80 pounds and my blood pressure and cholesterol are both perfectly normal."

Bruce Howard
San Francisco, California

To Be Healthy, Eat Healthfully

The thought process behind *Eat for Health* differs from conventional diets. When I first developed my approach to superior nutrition, I started by asking, "What is the healthiest way to eat?" The method that you will find in this book is my answer, perfected over the years. The fact that it is also the most effective way to lose weight is a great bonus. Other diets and nutrition plans seem to be based on the premise, "How can we make a popular diet, and what type of gimmick or hook will sell books?" My primary goal in writing and teaching nutritional information has never been popularity or economic success. As a doctor, I have a duty to patients who rely on me for lifesaving advice. My goal is to be scientifically accurate and create the eating-style that is most effective for both weight loss and disease reversal, bar none. Superior nutrition is the answer.

One of the most radical adjustments you will have to make in following *Eat for Health* is forgetting what you consider a normal portion size. Typical portion sizes are far too small for this plan. Get ready to discover that eating much larger amounts of the right foods—high-nutrient foods—is the secret to long-term weight loss and great health. While your focus is on increasing your consumption of high-nutrient foods, you may find that you aren't as hungry for the other less healthful foods that you previously relied upon. When you reduce the consumption of these foods is up to you. The sooner that these foods are less present in your diet, the faster you will see dramatic results.

The first step towards achieving superior health in your life is eating healthfully. This means eating more healthful foods. It sounds simple, right? It's not a brilliant or original idea, but most people don't understand which foods are truly nutritious. Lots of people think a diet designed around pasta, chicken, and olive oil is health-promoting, but are these foods actually good for you? The answer is no, or at least not in the quantities that the average American consumes them. This is because none of these foods are rich in nutrients.

What makes a food healthful is how many nutrients it delivers to your body. In other words, for optimal health we must eat foods that are truly rich in nutrients, and in particular, foods that deliver the maximum nutrients in each calorie. This can be a strange concept for many people because they are accustomed to evaluating a food by analyzing how many calories, fat grams, or carbohydrates it has. Try to wipe those ingrained ideas from your mind. With this plan, your primary concern will be the nutrients in the foods you eat. However, to eat this way, we must first understand what nutrients are and which foods are the most nutrient-dense.

Discovering Nutrients

There are two kinds of nutrients: macronutrients and micronutrients. Macronutrients are protein, carbohydrate, and fat. They contain calories. Micronutrients are vitamins, minerals, and phytochemicals and are calorie-free. For ideal health, we need to consume both kinds of nutrients, but the American diet contains too many macronutrients and not enough micronutrients.

MACRONUTRIENTS = FAT, CARBOHYDRATE, AND PROTEIN

CONTAIN CALORIES

SHOULD LIMIT CONSUMPTION

•

MICRONUTRIENTS = VITAMINS, MINERALS, AND PHYTOCHEMICALS

DO NOT CONTAIN CALORIES

SHOULD INCREASE CONSUMPTION

Eating foods that are rich in micronutrients is essential to achieving optimal health. A micronutrient-heavy diet supplies your body with 14 different vitamins, 25 different minerals, and more than 10,000 phytochemicals, which are plant-based chemicals that have profound effects on human cell function and the immune system. Foods that are naturally rich in these nutrients are also rich in fiber and water and are naturally low in calories, meaning they have a low caloric density. These low-calorie, high-nutrient foods provide the ingredients that enable your body's self-healing and self-repairing mechanisms. They are nature's contribution to your health turnaround!

In addition to eating more of these micronutrient-rich foods, we need to eat less of the macronutrients. Every nutritional scientist in the world agrees that moderate caloric restriction slows the aging process, prevents the development of chronic diseases, and extends lifespan. This has been tested in every species of animal, including primates. There is no controversy; Americans are eating themselves to death with too many calories. To change this we must do three things:

❶ EAT LESS FAT

❷ EAT LESS PROTEIN

❸ EAT LESS CARBOHYDRATE

Although these reductions will be part of our focus, this program is not primarily about calorie restriction. Simply trying to reduce calories is called dieting, and dieting doesn't work. The reason this program is so successful is because over time, without even trying or noticing it, you will prefer to eat fewer calories. I know that can sound unlikely. Many people think, "Not me," "My body doesn't work that way," or, "It will be a real struggle for me." However, if you follow the plan, it will happen instinctually. I have seen it happen to hundreds of my patients, with all kinds of different backgrounds and eating histories, and I promise, it can happen for you too.

This is the secret to nutritarian eating: achieve superior health by eating more nutrient-rich foods and less high-calorie, low-nutrient foods. **It works because the more high-nutrient food you consume, the less low-nutrient food you desire.** Since the desire for these unhealthy foods will naturally diminish, this program is fundamentally about learning how to enjoy eating more high-nutrient food.

Foods are nutrient dense when they contain a high level of micronutrients per calorie. Vegetables win the award for the most nutrient-dense foods on the planet. As you move forward in your quest for nutritional excellence, you will learn to eat more and more vegetables. Vegetables have the most powerful association with protection from heart disease and cancer because they contain the most nutrients per calorie. A year-round consumption of high-nutrient, plant-based foods is the secret to obtaining superior health and your ideal weight. The recipes provided at the end of this book will show you new and delicious ways to include many more vegetables in your daily menus.

Understanding the Nutritarian Diet-style

Vegetables and other high-nutrient foods are the cornerstones of *Eat for Health*, but this is not a book about becoming a strict vegetarian. Instead, this eating style is easily described with a word I coined:

NUTRITARIAN
A PERSON WHO STRIVES FOR MORE MICRONUTRIENTS PER CALORIE IN THEIR DIET-STYLE AND WHO AVOIDS UNHEALTHY FOOD CHOICES.

The nutritarian way to health, longevity, and dieting differentiates itself from flexitarian or vegetarian paths because the label of the eating-style is not defined merely by the amount, frequency, or lack of animal products. Instead, it is defined by the attention to consuming lots of high-nutrient, healthful foods such as green vegetables, berries, and seeds. A nutritarian usually eats fewer animal products than conventional eaters, but may or may not be a vegetarian or vegan. The eating-style is also distinguished by the limitation in the consumption of sugar, other sweeteners, white flour, refined oils, and processed foods in general.

I advocate a nutritarian eating-style. It affords many benefits for the individual and society in general by encouraging more people to take better care of their health through dietary improvements. To a degree, most people have some idea that eating better and eating more nutrient-rich foods will benefit them, but they just don't have the information to know what those foods are and to recognize the benefits and obstacles to adopting a healthful diet. Most likely you already are a nutritarian to some degree. This program will just make it easier for you to crystallize the eating-style you need to accomplish your goals.

Healthy Food Choices Are at Your Door

Historically, a year-round diet that included lots of vegetables and fruits simply wasn't possible. People were limited to foods that were grown locally and seasonally and a diet based on grains that could be stored for long periods.

It is always growing season somewhere. Today, improvements in transportation and refrigeration have made it possible to move and store fresh foods from around the globe. This has given us year-round access to the healthiest and most nutrient-dense foods and an unprecedented opportunity to achieve and maintain superior health.

Our understanding of the importance of these foods is also very recent. In the last 50 years there have been over 10,000 scientific studies showing the value of consuming high-nutrient plant foods. Here are a few critical points from these studies:

- Plants contain three classes of micronutrients that are critical for our health: vitamins, minerals, and phytochemicals. The finding of thousands of phytochemical compounds in natural plant foods is the most significant discovery in nutritional science in this century. We have learned these nutrients are essential for a highly effective immune system and protection from the common diseases of aging.

- A plant-based diet that is rich in colorful vegetables and fruits, such as this one, allows you to eat more food. With so many high-nutrient foods permitted in an unlimited quantity*, it makes it easy to eat until you're satisfied and still lose weight, without the need to count calories or restrict portions.

  * *without overeating*

- Increasing micronutrients and reducing calories enables the body to receive an assortment of protective health benefits and defy the aging process. In essence, these studies have shown that there is a way to extend life and delay the onset of aging, allowing you to live better and more healthfully in your later years.

Fifty years of scientific studies indicate that most diseases seen in modern countries, as well as the leading causes of death, are the result of dietary and lifestyle choices. Scientists have determined that inadequate consumption of plant-derived nutrients results in cellular toxicity, DNA damage, and immune system dysfunction. This, in turn, leads to increased susceptibility to infections, allergies, and even the development of cancer.

There is a way to eat that helps prevent these health problems and satisfies your hunger with fewer calories. A diet rich in high-nutrient plant foods is the most effective way to reduce your food cravings. As your level of micronutrients increases—by consuming greater amounts of high-nutrient foods—your appetite will naturally decrease. The result is that you will become healthier and will look and feel young well into your later years. There is no reason for anyone to develop heart disease, strokes, Type II diabetes or dementia. To prevent and reverse these and most of the chronic diseases in our modern world, you don't need instructions from a doctor's prescription pad. The prescription is nutrition.

Unhealthful Food Choices

Many people suffer from medical ailments because they were never taught about their bodies' nutritional requirements. As a country, we eat entirely too many low-nutrient foods, which deliver too many calories and not enough nutrients. When our nutrient deprived bodies then crave more food, the easy availability of calorie-rich, low nutrient foods enables us to eat ourselves to death. A diet based on milk, meats, cheese, pasta, bread, fried foods, and sugar-filled snacks and drinks lays the groundwork for obesity, cancer, heart disease, diabetes, digestive disorders, and autoimmune illnesses.

THE FOODS I JUST MENTIONED ARE HARMFUL IN THREE WAYS.

1) They are high in disease-promoting substances that undermine our health.

2) The more unhealthful foods you eat, the fewer health promoting, plant-based foods you will include in your diet.

3) Consuming calories that are lacking antioxidant vitamins and phytochemicals leads to a build-up of waste products in your cells because your body can't remove normal cellular wastes without nutrients. The cells don't have the raw materials needed for optimal or normal function. The lack of some substances and the excess of others ages us prematurely and causes disease.

Foods such as chips, cookies, bread, and pasta lose a dramatic amount of their nutrients in the refinement process. In addition to being nutrient poor, processed foods contain elements that contribute to our health problems: salt, chemical food additives, trans fats, MSG, sodium nitrate, and other unhealthful ingredients. The process that browns foods and turns a grain into a baked flake of chip also creates acrylamides, carcinogens that make foods even more harmful.

By contrast, unrefined plant foods, including vegetables, beans, nuts, seeds, and fruits, are the most nutrient-dense foods. Unfortunately, the average American consumes less than 7 percent of his or her calories from these foods. People who eat according to my guidelines however, consume over 70-90 percent of their calories from unrefined plant foods. By increasing the amount of nutrient-dense food you consume, you are directly influencing your body's chance to thrive.

CHAPTER THREE

THE POWER OF MICRONUTRIENTS

The Fountain of Youth

All the different types of nutrients are vital to achieving and maintaining superior nutrition and optimal health; however, phytochemicals hold a special, elite place in the nutritional landscape. When consistently consumed in sufficient quantities and varieties, phytochemicals become super-nutrients in your body. They work together to detoxify cancer-causing compounds, deactivate free radicals, protect against radiation damage, and enable DNA repair mechanisms.[19] When altered or broken strands of DNA are repaired, you are less likely to develop cancer later in life. I've made an acronym to make it easy to remember the super foods that offer the most protection against disease: **G-BOMBS**, which stands for **G**reens, **B**eans, **O**nions, **M**ushrooms, **B**erries and **S**eeds. More details about these superfoods can be found in my *New York Times* best-selling book, *Super Immunity*.

Consuming phytochemicals is not optional. They are essential in human immune-system defenses. Without a wide variety and sufficient amount of phytochemicals from unprocessed plant foods, cells age more rapidly and do not retain their innate ability to remove and detoxify waste products and toxic compounds. Low levels of phytochemicals in our modern diet are largely responsible for the common diseases seen with aging, especially cancer and heart disease. These are diseases caused by nutritional ignorance and in many cases, can be prevented. Approximately 85 percent of our population suffers from and eventually dies of heart disease, strokes, and cancer. This is extremely high compared to other populations around the world and at earlier points in human history.

Let's take heart disease as an example. Heart attacks are extremely rare occurrences in populations that eat a diet rich in protective phytochemicals, such as the Okinawans of Japan, but are omnipresent in populations, such as ours, that eat a diet low in protective nutrients.[20] Compelling data from numerous population and interventional studies shows that a natural, plant-based diet rich in antioxidants and phytochemicals will prevent, arrest, and even reverse heart disease.[21] With what we know about heart disease causation, practically no one needs to die of heart disease today.

Only via superior nutrition can you attack all the invisible, but potentially dangerous plaque throughout your coronary arteries. Unlike surgery and angioplasty, the dietary approach addressed in this book does not merely treat a small segment of your heart. It rejuvenates all your blood vessels and protects your entire body against heart attacks, strokes, venous thrombosis and pulmonary embolisms, peripheral vascular disease, and vascular dementia.

To receive the benefits of superior nutrition, however, you must actually eat well. Many people believe they can meet all of their nutrient needs by taking supplements. However, supplements can't match or duplicate all the protective, strengthening elements of real fruits and vegetables. There are too many unknown and undiscovered factors in these natural foods. There are more than 10,000 identified phytochemicals, with more being discovered all the time. Only by eating a diet rich in whole foods can we assure ourselves of obtaining a full symphony of these disease-protecting, anti-aging nutrients. Supplements can be useful in delivering micronutrients found in foods that would be very difficult to incorporate into our diet, such as fatty fish. This is why the word supplement is a good one: the pill is supplemental to a healthy diet, not a replacement for it.

Our bodies were designed to make use of thousands of plant compounds. When these necessary compounds are missing, we might survive because our bodies are adaptable, but we pay a price. Without them, we lose our powerful potential for wellness. Chronic diseases often develop, and we are robbed of living to our fullest potential in good physical, emotional, and mental health. Ultimately, we are what we eat. We get the materials to build our cells from our diet because food provides the raw materials that our bodies use to create tissue and to function at a high level. Consumption of healthy foods leads to disease resistance; consumption of unhealthy foods makes us disease-prone.

Eating right enables you to feel your best everyday. You may still get sick from a virus, but your body will be in a far better position to defend itself and make a quick and complete recovery. Optimal nutrition enables you to work better, play better, and maintain your youthful vigor as you age gracefully.

Micronutrient Density

For optimal health, you need to eat foods that are high in micronutrients per calorie. This important nutritional concept can be presented by a simple mathematical formula, which I call my health equation.

DR. FUHRMAN'S HEALTH EQUATION:

$$H = N/C$$

HEALTH = NUTRIENTS/CALORIES

Your future Health (H) will increase as your Nutrient (N)* to Calorie (C) ratio increases.

*Nutrient (N) refers to *micro*nutrients

Your health is dependent on the nutrient-per-calorie density of your diet (micronutrients consumed divided by calories consumed). This straightforward mathematical formula is the basis of nutritional science and nutritional healing. For you to build and maintain excellent health, your diet must be micronutrient rich, and you must not overeat on calories or macronutrients. The nutrient density in your body's tissues is proportional to the nutrient density of your diet. Choose foods and design your diet with this equation in mind. Consume more foods with a high nutrient-per-calorie density and less foods with a low nutrient-per-calorie density. Make every calorie count.

How do you know which foods have the highest nutrient-per-calorie density? To answer this question, I have ranked the nutrient density of many common foods in the table below using my Aggregate Nutrient Density Index, or ANDI. This Index assigns a score to a variety of foods based on how many nutrients they deliver to your body for each calorie consumed. Each of the food scores is out of a possible 1000 based on the nutrients per calorie equation. Food labels, when they are required at all, list only a few nutrients, but my scores are based on twenty-eight important micronutrients plus other phytochemicals.

ANDI scores let you quickly see which foods promote the healthiest outcomes. That way, you can evaluate the quality of your current diet and get an idea of how much better it will be when you start adding high-nutrient foods (and eliminating low-nutrient ones). The scores are a simple way to help you identify and eat larger amounts of nutrient-dense foods. The higher the scores and the greater percentage of those foods in your diet, the better your health will be.

Because phytochemicals are largely unnamed and unmeasured, these ANDI rankings may underestimate the healthful properties of colorful, natural, plant foods compared to processed foods and animal products. One thing we do know about natural foods is this: The foods that contain the highest amount of known nutrients are the same foods that contain the most unknown nutrients. So, even though these scores may need to be revised somewhat as science uncovers new phytochemicals, they still represent a reasonable guide to understanding the value of the foods you eat.

NUTRIENT PER CALORIE DENSITY SCORES

Kale 1000

Collard Greens. 1000

Mustard Greens 1000

Watercress 1000

Swiss Chard 895

Bok Choy 865

Spinach. 707

Arugula 604

Romaine 510

Brussels Sprouts 490

Carrots 458

Cabbage 434

Broccoli 340

Cauliflower 315

Bell Peppers 265

Mushrooms 238

Asparagus. 205

Tomato 186

Strawberries 182

Sweet Potato. 181

Zucchini 164

Artichoke 145

Blueberries 132

Iceberg Lettuce 127

Milk, 1% 31

Walnuts. 30

Bananas 30

Whole Wheat Bread 30

Almonds 28

Avocado 28

Brown Rice 28

White Potato 28

Low Fat Plain Yogurt 28

Cashews. 27

Chicken Breast 24

Ground Beef, 85% lean. 21

Feta Cheese 20

White Bread. 17

    estimated ANDI without fortification. 9

White Pasta. 16

    estimated ANDI without fortification. 11

French Fries 12

Cheddar Cheese 11

Apple Juice 11

Olive Oil 10

Vanilla Ice Cream. 9

Corn Chips 7

Cola 1

For a complete guide of ANDI scores, read my *Nutritarian Handbook and Food Scoring Guide.*

Nutrient Scoring Method*

To determine the ANDI scores, an equal-calorie serving of each food was evaluated. The following nutrients were included in the evaluation: fiber, calcium, iron, magnesium, phosphorus, potassium, zinc, copper, manganese, selenium, vitamin A, beta carotene, alpha carotene, lycopene, lutein and zeaxanthin, vitamin E, vitamin C, thiamin, riboflavin, niacin, pantothenic acid, vitamin B6, folate, vitamin B12, choline, vitamin K, phytosterols, glucosinolates, angiogenesis inhibitors, organosulfides, aromatase inhibitors, resistant starch, resveratrol plus ORAC score. ORAC (Oxygen Radical Absorbance Capacity) is a measure of the antioxidant or radical scavenging capacity of a food. For consistency, nutrient quantities were converted from their typical measurement conventions (mg, mcg, IU) to a percentage of their Dietary Reference Intake (DRI). For nutrients that have no DRI, goals were established based on available research and current understanding of the benefits of these factors.

To make it easier to compare foods, the raw point totals were converted (multiplied by the same number) so that the highest ranking foods (leafy green vegetables) received a score of 1000, and the other foods received lower scores accordingly.

Knowing the Score

As expected, green vegetables win the prize and no other food is even close. No wonder green vegetables have the best association with lower rates of cancer and heart disease. While most people are eating the majority of their calories from foods with the lower scores, you can increase your consumption of high-scoring foods and dramatically improve and protect your health.

It is important to achieve micronutrient diversity, not just a high level of a few isolated micronutrients. Micronutrient adequacy means obtaining enough of all beneficial nutrients, not merely higher amounts of a select few, while other micronutrient needs go unfulfilled.

Eating a variety of plant foods is the key to achieving micronutrient diversity. Consider mushrooms to illustrate this concept. Mushrooms may not contain the highest amounts of vitamins and minerals, but they contain a significant amount of protective phytochemicals that are not found in other foods, such as aromatase inhibitors and angiogenesis inhibitors. A small amount of mushrooms in the diet adds more micronutrient diversity, even though they are not the highest scoring food when we add up all their micronutrients. Focus not only on the nutritional quality of what you eat, but also on the proper spectrum of foods that supply the full symphonic orchestra of human requirements. This means that certain plant foods such as onions, seeds, mushrooms, berries, beans, and tomatoes aid in achieving micronutrient quality and contribute to the numerator in my H=N/C equation, even though they might not have the most nutrients per calorie. The recipes and menus at the end of this book will help you achieve this goal.

In any of the levels of *Eat For Health*, there are some foods that you can eat in relatively unlimited quantities, the *ultimate foods* in terms of nutrient density and excellence. Memorize the categories below. If you can learn to make your recipes and meals mostly from the foods in these categories, you will be maximizing the nutrient density of your diet. You will protect yourself from illness and disease in the future and have the greatest chance of recovering your health if you are currently unhealthy.

HIGH-NUTRIENT FOODS THAT CAN BE EATEN IN NEARLY UNLIMITED QUANTITIES
(without overeating, of course):

LEAFY GREEN VEGETABLES
romaine lettuce, leaf lettuces, kale, collards, Swiss chard, mustard greens, spinach, bok choy, watercress

SOLID GREEN VEGETABLES
artichokes, asparagus, broccoli, brussels sprouts, cabbage, celery, cucumber, kohlrabi, okra, peas, green peppers, snow peas, string beans, zucchini

NON-GREEN, HIGH-NUTRIENT VEGETABLES
beets, eggplant, mushrooms, onions, tomatoes, peppers, garlic, leeks, cauliflower, squash, carrots

BEANS AND LEGUMES
red kidney beans, adzuki beans, chickpeas, pinto beans, edamame, navy beans, cannelloni beans, soybeans, lentils, white beans, lima beans, pigeon peas, black-eyed peas, black beans, split peas

FRESH FRUITS
apples, apricots, blackberries, blueberries, grapefruit, grapes, kiwis, mangoes, nectarines, all melons, oranges, peaches, pears, persimmons, pineapples, plums, raspberries, strawberries, tangerines

CHAPTER FOUR

WHAT'S ON YOUR PLATE?

Pyramid or Plate?

By now, you understand that the key component to *Eat For Health* is eating more vegetables, fruits, and other nutrient-rich foods. Let's divide foods into three types: animal products, processed foods, and unprocessed plant foods. *Eat For Health* dramatically reduces both animal products and processed foods in your diet and increases consumption of unprocessed plant foods, the most nutrient-rich foods on the planet. Even among the unprocessed plant foods, I encourage you to eat more of the most cancer-protective foods, such as greens, mushrooms and onions. Remember to use my easy acronym for these superfoods: **G-BOMBS**, which stands for the most beneficial foods: **Greens, Beans, Onions, Mushrooms, Berries and Seeds.** As a safety precaution, mushrooms should be consumed cooked, not raw.

Over the years, Americans became accustomed to seeing the United States Department of Agriculture (USDA) food pyramid, which was supposed to be a guide to healthful food choices. Unfortunately, the design of the food pyramid was always strongly influenced by social, business, and political concerns, not pure science. As a result, the USDA pyramid was never a reliable guide. This is one reason why so many Americans are confused about nutrition and plagued with obesity and preventable diseases. If you wanted to design a food pyramid that would actually help people, the base would consist of foods that should be consumed in the highest quantity, followed by foods that should be consumed regularly, followed by foods that should be consumed infrequently. The USDA pyramid didn't do this. In fact, its design encouraged people to regularly eat foods that should only be eaten rarely, if at all.

I developed a new pyramid. For superior health, we must eat more nutrient-rich foods and fewer low-nutrient, high-calorie foods. The top of my pyramid is composed of the foods lowest in nutrients, such as processed foods like chips and cookies. These are the foods that should be consumed very rarely if at all. The base is comprised of the nutrient-rich plant foods according to their nutrient composition and disease-protective properties.

When the nutritional landscape of America is shaped by nutrient density as represented in my pyramid, we will have dramatically extended our healthy life expectancy and will see health care costs plummet.

Dr. Fuhrman's Food Pyramid

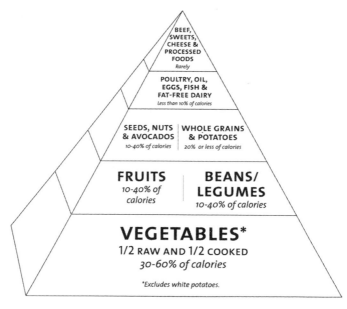

The USDA Food Pyramid has been replaced by their Choose My Plate icon. It does put more emphasis on the consumption of vegetables and fruit but it still has some fundamental flaws. Foods are still grouped in a way that does not make sense.

Meat, beans and nuts and seeds are in the same food group because they are considered protein-rich foods. However, while nuts, seeds and beans have been shown to reduce cholesterol levels and heart disease, meat is linked to increased risk. The USDA's My Plate would also lead you to believe that dairy products should be consumed on a daily basis. Including milk as its own prominent group implies that it is an essential part of a healthy diet, which is anything but the truth, especially considering the strong association of dairy with negative health consequences including several cancers. This plate offers little help for those really wanting to reduce their health risks.

USDA's MyPlate

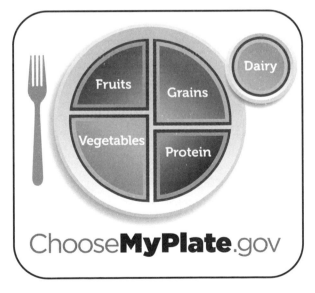

My Nutritarian Food Plate illustrates what your plate should really look like. It is comprised of the nutrient-rich plant foods according to their nutrient composition and disease-protective properties. The foods that are featured on my plate are raw and cooked vegetables, fruit, beans, nuts and seeds.

DR. FUHRMAN'S NUTRITARIAN FOOD PLATE©

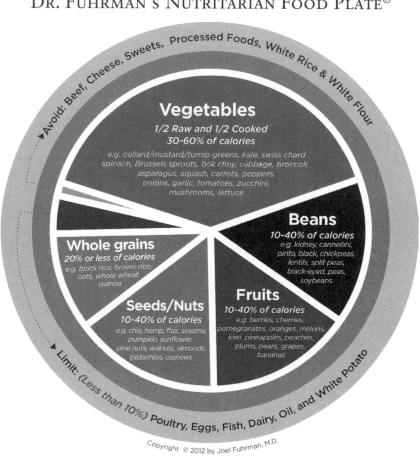

Copyright © 2012 by Joel Fuhrman, M.D.

The Dangers of Omission

Our society has evolved to a level of economic sophistication that allows us to eat ourselves to death. A diet centered on milk, cheese, pasta, bread, fried foods, sugar-filled snacks and drinks, lays the groundwork for obesity, cancer, heart disease, diabetes, and autoimmune illnesses. These foods certainly are harmful, but that is not the whole problem. Part of the problem is that we are not eating enough nutrient-rich foods.

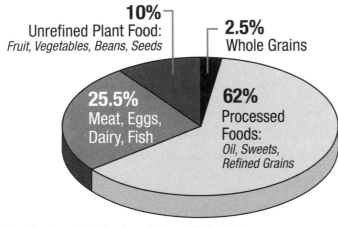

10%
Unrefined Plant Food:
Fruit, Vegetables, Beans, Seeds

2.5%
Whole Grains

25.5%
Meat, Eggs,
Dairy, Fish

62%
Processed
Foods:
*Oil, Sweets,
Refined Grains*

United States Department of Agriculture Economics Research Service, 2005.
http://www.ers.usda.gov/Data/FoodConsumption/FoodGuideIndex.htm#calories

America's Food Consumption Pie

As this chart shows, when you evaluate the Standard American Diet (SAD), you find that the calories coming from phytochemical-rich foods, such as fresh fruit, vegetables, beans, raw nuts, and seeds, are less than 13 percent of the total caloric intake. This dangerously low intake of unrefined plant foods is what guarantees weakened immunity to disease, frequent illnesses, and a shorter life expectancy. We will never win the war on cancer, heart disease, diabetes, autoimmune diseases, and other degenerative illnesses unless we address this deficiency. The American diet has spread all over the world, bringing with it heart disease, cancer, and obesity, but studies still show that in the populations that eat more fruits and vegetables, the incidence of death from these diseases is dramatically lower.[22]

Most health authorities today are in agreement that we should add more servings of fruits and vegetables to our diet. I disagree somewhat. Thinking about our diet in this fashion doesn't adequately address the problem. Instead of adding protective fruits, vegetables, beans, and nuts to a disease-causing diet, we must make **these foods the main focus of the diet.** This is what makes my high nutrient approach different. Once we make nutrient-rich vegetables, fruits, beans and nuts the caloric foundation of the diet, then maybe we can safely add a few small servings of lower-nutrient foods like animal products.

Foods to Die For

Most Americans are not in good health, thanks to the standard, low-nutrient diet in this country. The risk of developing high blood pressure, diabetes and heart disease, is extremely high for all people who eat this way. So is the risk of cardiovascular related premature death. Look at these statistics:

- The lifetime risk for developing hypertension (high blood pressure) is over 90 percent.[23]

- High blood pressure has climbed 30 percent over the past decade.

- Cardiovascular disease (CVD) is an enormous health care burden and is responsible for approximately 40 percent of all U.S. deaths annually.[24]

There's nothing pre-programmed in the human genome that says as people get old they automatically get fat and have high blood pressure. They develop high blood pressure because their diets are calorie-rich and nutrient-poor. High blood pressure and heart disease are not the consequences of aging. They are the result of the slow insidious damage created from years and years of poor dietary choices.

Processed foods, too much salt, and lack of physical exercise all contribute to the problem. Then people are given prescription drugs that allow them to continue their disease-causing habits while gaining a false sense of security. If you eat like other Americans, you will either have a heart attack and die when you are young, or you will inevitably develop high blood pressure and then be at high risk for either a heart attack or stroke when you get older. Populations around the world who live and eat differently have elderly members who are free of high blood pressure.[25] These diseases have known nutritional causes, and you never need to suffer from them.

Today, two in five Americans are obese, and the three out of five Americans who are not obese are significantly overweight. We are in worse shape today, with heavier bodies and thicker waistlines, than at any time in human history. At the same time, scientists have learned that our waistlines and our weight are the most critical factors governing our health and lifespan. In spite of an overwhelming amount of scientific evidence, people are still dying prematurely and living poor quality lives plagued by sickness and disability. Heart disease, diabetes, and most cancers are preventable, but prevention requires change. It sounds simple, and it can be simple if you have an open mind and if you let knowledge, rather than habits and emotions, guide you.

Learn from Your Elders

Our bodies are designed to live long, healthy lives, free from the common diseases of aging. However, years of abuse leaves its toll. If water runs over a waterfall and pounds into a rock at high speed, it wears down and eventually splits the rock in two. It was not aging that broke the rock; it was the water that took its toll on it after many thousands of years. Likewise, we develop hardening of the arteries, high blood pressure, heart disease, dementia, and other debilitating conditions from our dietary follies that take their toll over many years of nutritional self-abuse. These common ailments are not the consequence of aging. They are earned.

Researchers have found that people who exceed 100 years in age can be remarkably disease-free. Boston and Harvard University Scientists involved with the New England Centenarian Study (NECS) have been studying many long-lived individuals.

Among other factors, they tracked genetics, physical and mental health, and lifestyle habits. They found that long-lived people generally do not have the age-associated medical conditions that develop and curtail enjoyment of life at an early age. In other words, living healthfully goes hand in hand with living longer. These people, who are now past 100, did not have the advantage of the scientific information that we have today. For the majority of their lives, they did not have access to the healthiest foods. The question is, how did they do it, and what skills can we learn from these super seniors?

For starters, none of these centenarians were overweight. To achieve your maximum health potential you must manage your weight. **You can literally stretch your lifespan by shrinking your waistline.** Developing a high-nutrient diet and maintaining a stable, lower weight is the most powerful anti-aging weapon in your arsenal. However, we also must consider evidence that nutritional deficiencies have been shown to cause disease and disability. The goal is to maintain a high or adequate nutrient intake and ensure that no deficiencies exist, while making sure we do not consume excess calories. Yet again, the secret is incorporating large amounts of high-nutrient, low-calorie foods into your diet.

When looking at long-lived, elderly people within a society like ours, in which people eat similarly and the average age of death is about 78, we are selecting individuals with favorable genetics. Scientific studies don't tell us much because most of our population eats the standard (disease-causing) diet. When we look at outcomes, they merely reflect genetic influences, not vast differences in the consumption of micronutrients. It would be more revealing if we could look at an entire population that has an average lifespan over the age of ninety and see what the population did to achieve that. John Robbins' book, *Healthy At 100*, reviewed the lifestyles of the longest-lived populations around the globe in recent world history. The top three societies were the Abkhasia in the Caucasus region south of Russia, the Vilcabamba in the Andes of South America, and the Hunza in Central Asia. These isolated cultures not only have populations with very long average lives, but their elderly are also in excellent health, free of common diseases seen in our modern world.

The diets in all of these ultra long-lived societies contain at least 90 percent of calories from unrefined foods: high-nutrient fruits, vegetables, beans, nuts, and seeds. Animal products are a much smaller part of the equation, ranging between 1-10 percent of calories. These societies consist of physically active people who grow most of their own food and eat mostly fresh vegetables and fruits. These healthy societies reveal that, in addition to being slim, there are other important factors that super-seniors share:

- They consume the majority of calories from fresh produce.

- They have an optimistic outlook on life.

- They maintain a social circle of friends.

- They stay physically active.

Analyzing the results of these studies in terms of diet, it seems clear that an eating-style that promotes dramatic increases in lifespan and protects against later-life diseases includes:

❶ HIGH-NUTRIENT FOODS

❷ NO EXCESS CALORIES

❸ NO NUTRIENT DEFICIENCIES

The greater the amount and variety of nutrients, especially antioxidants and phytochemicals, you consume, the better your immune function and resistance to disease. You can see these benefits at any age. I have elderly patients that have been coming to see me for more than 10 years, and I have seen their blood-pressure and cholesterol readings fall gradually over the ten-year period while they were following my dietary suggestions. Rather than seeing the gradual rise in blood pressure and cholesterol with age, I have observed the opposite. After many years, they eventually reach the low systolic blood pressures we commonly see in children. The point is that aging is not the cause of high blood pressure; it is the time spent eating the conventional American diet that takes its toll.

To increase your chances of becoming one of those super-seniors, you should eat lots of whole foods that are naturally rich in protective nutrients. Take advantage of the fresh produce shipped all over the country. Never before in human history has year-round access to such high-quality food been available to such a large population. Eating high-nutrient foods can allow more people to survive into their hundreds and enjoy optimal health.

Even if your genetic potential does not match most of these super-seniors, you can still have the opportunity to live a long, healthy life because you can choose to eat high on the nutrient-density line. Nutrition and other lifestyle factors that you choose are more significant determinants of your health than genetics.

Virtually all disease is the result of the interaction of genetics and modifiable environmental and behavioral factors. Rarely does a single gene variant lead to the development of disease. Common diseases such as cancer, heart disease, and diabetes result from the complex interplay of genes and environment and cannot be classified as only genetic or environmental. The reality is that both genetics and the environment contribute to disease, and the biggest component of environmental causation is diet.

A good example is breast cancer. Less than one percent of women living in rural China get breast cancer, whereas 18 percent of American women eventually suffer with the disease. Yet when Asian women immigrate to America and adopt the richer American diet, which is higher in calories and animal products and lower in vegetables, they suffer the same breast cancer rates as other Americans.[26] Genes interact with environmental factors to influence an individual's susceptibility to disease. When these environmental promoters are not present, the disease simply does not exist.

Despite medical advances, 85 percent of Americans will still die from heart disease, cancer, or diabetes. The real key to longevity is not better treatment; it is prevention. In comparison with our sickly nation, people who survive past 100 years are remarkably disease-free. They are generally physically active, independent, and socially connected. They are not the feeble stereotypes that we often associate with getting old. This is not merely about living longer; it is also about staying younger and healthier into our later years, so life can be enjoyed to its fullest. Once you grasp the possibilities, your entire way of thinking will change. You do not have to be a victim. You can experience a long, disease-free life!

CHAPTER FIVE

EXERCISES WITH FOOD: DIETARY WARM UPS

While you are learning about the *Eat For Health* plan, I encourage you to do some Dietary Warm Ups to start getting you in shape for your new diet style. It is important that you think of these exercises in the same way that you think of exercises at the gym. When you go to the gym, you don't expect to suddenly build muscle; that takes time. You may not even enjoy going when you first start out. The excitement comes later, when you see your body starting to change.

You can apply this same way of thinking to your new way of eating. The dietary exercises that follow will begin to increase your appreciation of natural whole foods. The foods may seem foreign at first, and you may not experience the same enjoyment that you are accustomed to. But that is expected. As with exercise, the reward comes later, when you begin to develop a taste for new foods and start to see your body changing. The exercises expose your palate to new flavors and textures, which can take time to get used to. Some people mistakenly conclude that the food will never taste good. A better way of thinking about it is that the tastes and textures are unfamiliar, and they will take a little time to get used to. That is why I designed these exercises. Start small and progress at your own speed. Don't do too much too fast, but do your exercises consistently.

EXERCISE 1

The first exercise is to eat one-half pound of cut up raw vegetables and one-half pound of low-calorie fruits each day. This is not that much food. You should do this exercise at the same time each day. I recommend eating the fruit at breakfast and the raw vegetables in the afternoon before dinner. The important thing is to do the exercise close to mealtime and not when you have a full stomach. You should feel like eating. Remember not to eat too heavily at lunch, so that you are hungry enough later in the afternoon, before dinner, to eat your raw vegetables. The goal of this exercise is to eat a comfortable amount of raw vegetables, including tomatoes, red pepper, carrots, broccoli spears, celery, snow pea pods, and zucchini, and fruits including fresh berries, cantaloupe, kiwi, and apple slices. Over time, see if you can comfortably increase the volume of food.

After eating all these raw vegetables and fruits, you may decide to eat less at dinner because you feel too full, but let that decision come naturally. Try not to overeat, but don't restrict yourself either. Eat the amount that feels comfortable, and try to stop eating before you feel full. Stop when you're satisfied. Finding the difference between satisfied and full is an important step in becoming a healthy eater.

EXERCISE 2

The second exercise can be done at the same time as the first. While you are eating those fruits and vegetables during the day, chew each mouthful until every piece of food is liquefied. This will take a considerable amount of time and will feel very different from how you are used to eating, but how you eat is very important. Eating slowly is the only way to obtain all the nutrients from a food. You can access the full nutrient load by breaking open every single plant cell. Eating this way will also exercise your jaw and help you develop healthier gums and teeth. Remember: chew, chew, chew.

The most important element of these exercises is performing them every single day. Doing them daily will not only increase your enjoyment of healthy foods, but it will also help you lose weight. In the beginning, you may continue eating some foods from your traditional diet, although you will probably be eating a lot less of them. Over time, you will be more comfortable eliminating your unhealthy food choices and replacing them with healthful ones because your palate will desire them. Let this process happen at its own pace. Do not do these exercises instead of eating a meal, especially in this beginning stage.

A skill is a developed talent or ability, and being healthy is the result of several skills. The difficulty comes when you try to be proficient in all of those skills at once. Enjoying the taste of nutrient-dense food is a skill. Giving up old foods that you love in favor of new foods that you don't like requires multiple skills. These exercises isolate and target specific skill sets. They will help you avoid the anxiety that many feel when they give up their old way of eating all of a sudden. The method that I have developed is a purposeful and effective way to assist you in your transition to preferring a healthy approach to eating.

WARM UP GOALS

- Have at least three fresh fruits with your breakfast.

- Eat a large salad or raw vegetables as part of your dinner every night, and chew thoroughly

Some people can jump right in and immediately switch to the ideal high-nutrient way of eating. I consider the ideal version of this diet to be one that contains at least 90 percent of calories from the healthiest foods; vegetables, fruits, beans, raw nuts, seeds, avocados, and whole grains. For some people, this change may feel too dramatic. It is not always easy to give up foods that you love and replace them with unfamiliar ones. Also, some people experience uncomfortable physical or mental symptoms when making the change. The modified approach that you are learning here works in sync with your brain so that you won't feel withdrawal or deprivation.

Don't be afraid to eat healthful foods. The focus here is on eating more, not less. The more raw and cooked green vegetables you consume, the less space you will have to eat high-calorie, low-nutrient foods. As the illustration below demonstrates, you will fill a sizeable volume of space in your stomach with a very small number of calories. This will help you comfortably cut the number of calories that you eat each day. This is very much like gastric bypass surgery without the surgery.

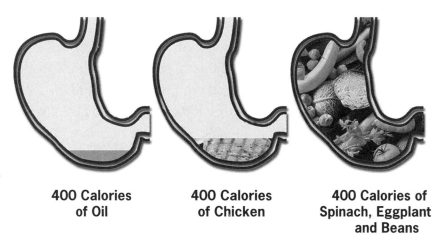

400 Calories of Oil   **400 Calories of Chicken**   **400 Calories of Spinach, Eggplant and Beans**

Adjust the amount of raw vegetables you eat to what your body will comfortably tolerate. If you experience uncomfortable gas, cut back a little on raw vegetables and beans. Don't remove these foods, because the goal is to let the body adjust the timing and secretion of its digestive enzymes and peristalsis to accommodate this healthy, more natural diet-style. You should be able to increase the amount of raw vegetables gradually without a problem. Don't forget to concentrate on chewing more thoroughly, because that may solve the problem. It can take time for your digestive system to build up the capacity to digest raw, whole foods, especially after a lifetime of eating a low-fiber diet.

There is another benefit to chewing well. Eating too quickly encourages overeating and can tax the digestive system. It takes about fifteen minutes for your brain to realize that your stomach is full. If you eat too fast, your body won't have enough time to tell you when it's full. You will end up eating more than you really need. Slow down, thoroughly chew your food, and enjoy the experience of eating.

CHAPTER SIX

GET INSIDE YOUR HEAD

"When I was 12, my family moved from Nebraska to Texas. I was miserable after the move and comforted myself with food. Eating for comfort became a familiar pattern, and I struggled with my weight, going on and off diets until I turned 40. At that point, I just gave up trying to be thin. I had enough failures and struggles. It seemed less stressful to accept being fat forever than to keep failing. I told myself that it was reality, like knowing that I can't reverse the clock and be 20 again. After that, I continued to gain about eight pounds each year until I was over 200 pounds. Then a friend recommended Dr. Fuhrman's book, *Eat To Live*. I was skeptical. I had tried many other programs, and they were all about meagerness and phony substitutes. I could never resign myself to that. I enjoy tasting food and I like to eat plenty of it, but I read Eat to Live and started trying the program slowly, just as Dr. Fuhrman recommends. I was shocked. The program was all about abundance, which was quite a change! What made the difference for me were two main things: the information about how the body uses nutrients, and trying it and seeing that it was not only doable, but also enjoyable.

I thought it would be impossible to give up my favorite foods: pasta, bread, butter, olive oil, and cheese. It was hard at first, but I made the best of it and ate lots of the nutrient-dense foods. I kept eating that way, and, after about six weeks, I realized that I never really missed those foods. It was then that I thought, "This works! I'm eating a lot of food, not feeling deprived and losing weight. I can do this!" For the first time ever, I allowed myself to say, "I'm not going to be fat always. I will be a slim, healthy person!" In my younger years I thought something magical would happen to make me slim. With this plan, I know that it's not magic. I can control it! This is for real and I'm doing it"

Elizabeth Jeffery
Minneapolis, Minnesota

Steps to a Healthful Diet

It is a sad fact that what we hear about nutrition and dieting from TV, radio, newspapers, diet books and even most of the scientific research community is thoroughly confusing. Almost every article or show on the topic discusses some magic food, supplement, metabolism booster, or fat-carbohydrate-protein ratio that can solve all of your weight problems. Research articles continue to test diets that are low in fat, high in fat, low in carbohydrates, and high in carbohydrates, and the media continues to report on them as though they represented some important new information. But trying to micromanage carbohydrate, fat or protein intake will not increase your health and longevity. This sort of dieting only encourages temporary fluctuations in calorie intake, leading to non-sustained changes in body weight, often called yo-yo dieting. These diets are bad for your health because it is not healthy to lose and gain weight over and over. What these studies actually show is that diets that don't address nutrient quality do not work.

There is no magical ratio of fat, carbohydrate, or protein that will lead you to your ideal weight and superior health. Rather, science has shown that only substantial changes in the quality of the nutrients you eat (with special attention given to micronutrients) can positively influence your body in terms of health, caloric drives, and weight. You need to learn and adopt a new way of living that will improve your quality of life for years to come. We now have the knowledge to maximize nutrition to the point where genetic predispositions will not have the chance to express themselves.

The incredible increase in overweight individuals, obesity, diabetes, and heart disease in the last century did not occur because people have changed their genes. It occurred because they changed their diets. The toxic food environment that pervades every city and town can make it difficult for people to find or accept the path back to healthful eating. However, by reading this book and adopting my nutritarian diet-style, you are setting yourself apart. You are beginning to create a new environment for yourself that allows your body to thrive, maximize its genetic potential and enhance its disease-protective capacity. If everyone would create that environment for themselves, we would achieve dramatic increases in healthy life expectancy and longevity.

Unlike trendy diets focused on one food or a type of food, this high-nutrient diet requires that you use your mind to evaluate all aspects of the way you eat. To be successful in achieving a healthful diet for yourself, you must accomplish the following:

❶ REPROGRAM YOUR THINKING AND TASTES TO PREFER MICRONUTRIENT-RICH FOODS.

❷ ELIMINATE ADDICTIVE HUNGER SYMPTOMS THAT LEAD TO OVEREATING BY MAKING MICRONUTRIENT-RICH FOODS THE FOUNDATION OF YOUR DIET

❸ LIMIT UNHEALTHFUL FOODS IN YOUR DAILY DIET.

As you increase your intake of high-nutrient food, you will desire unhealthful, low-nutrient food less and less. As you progress through this book, you will continue to limit your intake of these foods, including animal products, and refined, processed foods such as white flour and sugar. In the next chapters, we will discuss managing your hunger and ensuring you don't over-consume calories. We will focus on how you think about food and how you can reprogram your tastes.

While it is important to understand and think about each of these steps, it's also important to realize that they do not exist independently. We need to eat less fat, protein, and carbohydrates, the only three sources of calories in food. Obviously, we need calories, but we want to make sure that when we do consume them, the fat, protein, and carbohydrates that we choose to eat are in foods that are as micronutrient dense as possible. The healthiest way to eat, and the way to learn to naturally and automatically desire fewer calories, is to consistently consume high-nutrient meals. When you understand and follow these principles, you will be amazed at how easy and simple it is to achieve your ideal weight and health!

Your Powerful Mind

My book, *Eat To Live*, was written to help the overweight person recover their health and lose their stubborn, excess weight by following the most healthful and most effective diet.

Eat for Health was written for everyone, whether you have weight to lose or not. It features the same principles as *Eat to Live* but illustrates three levels of healthful eating. Many people need to make dramatic changes in the way they think before they can be asked to change the way they eat. They also need to approach the changes gradually, versus all at once. The three levels presented here give you the opportunity to make the changes more gradually. We are all born with an innate desire to not only survive but to thrive. Somewhere along the line, we have forgotten that fundamental imperative and have picked up so many bad habits that it can take some time to adjust.

In our modern society, we have lost touch with the instincts that lead us to healthful, life-sustaining behaviors. We graduate from elementary school, high school, college, and even graduate school and don't learn the one most important thing we should know: how to protect our health. Consider that 38 percent of our population dies of heart disease and strokes. That number is a deeper tragedy because they are needless and avoidable deaths. The solution is readily available, but few are aware of it.

For many, even when the information is presented to them, the fear of change and loss of pleasure forces them to close their eyes to it. In a perfect world, all people would live healthfully, get enough sleep, exercise, and eat the high-nutrient diet that would best protect their precious health. This seems almost impossible because most people believe that the change would be too hard. For them, my approach seems counter intuitive. It is radically different from what they are used to, and they think it would be too difficult, so they dismiss it. The mountain of supporting scientific evidence is not sufficiently persuasive. They need something more than just cold science to inspire them. Some people are so addicted to their present, dangerous diet that they would prefer death to change.

My goal is to uncover and address all the conscious and subconscious impediments you might face.

Conflicting Messages

The principal reason why people have difficulty adopting a healthful diet is because they have internal conflict. One part of them wants to be healthy, while another wants to do something that is not healthful, usually something that gives them pleasure in the moment, like eating a pint of ice cream. While you hold the carton and spoon in your hands, you want to eat the ice cream. In the larger perspective, you want to be healthy and lead a long, productive life. This book will help you rectify those two desires.

Adopting a healthful lifestyle generally requires change on many levels. Each level is controlled by a different region of the brain, and each level is like a different frequency or radio channel. As a result, you need to work on all aspects of yourself until being healthy and maintaining an ideal weight comes naturally. My goal is to help you to adopt a healthy set of core beliefs and automatic responses so that eventually you will follow a healthy lifestyle without any conscious effort. The process is not about strengthening your will-power, calorie-counting or any other gimmick.

To achieve permanent success in the health and weight loss arena, we have to consider the complexity of human nature. We are physical, emotional and social beings. We must consider all these factors. If we don't, it will increase the chance that we will reject health-giving information as too difficult, in spite of our interest in it. This is a physical manifestation of a subconscious process. Our brains are designed to dim awareness to information that causes us anxiety.

For most people, the idea of overhauling the way they think about food and the way they eat is a source of anxiety. Plus, unhealthful foods are a slow-working poison. Many ailments related to the foods people eat take years to develop, and the only visible issue for most people is their excess weight. Studies have shown that most overweight people routinely underestimate the extent of their obesity and do not see themselves as that overweight. Consequently, it is not too difficult to imagine how so many people can ignore the evidence. They don't see what it has to do with them. This is especially true for people who have low self-esteem.

Addressing Your Self-Worth

The objection of those unwilling to change their diet can sometimes have very little to do with the food. It is often the direct result of low self-esteem, which makes them vulnerable to negative peer pressure, addictions, and emotional over-eating. Some may fear appearing different from others, and they think changing the way they eat will result in a loss of social status. This is a subconscious perception, but some people are unknowingly governed by it. Others overeat to raise dopamine production in the brain, so that they can dull the frustration and pain of life.

As social animals, our brains require certain hormones that are released when we have positive social interaction. Eliminate these interactions and the brain will seek out other ways to produce the hormones and receive stimulatory input. This is why people with strong social ties are far less likely to be drawn into compulsive over-eating and other addictive behaviors. Several studies have shown that overeating, like drug and alcohol abuse, leads to dopamine stimulation. For people who are dependent on dopamine surges and who lack the emotional fulfillment that can provide them, consumption of high-calorie foods gives the brain the surge it is looking for. Therefore, they are more compelled to engage in this stimulating or toxic eating behavior. Their beliefs about themselves set in motion a chain of chemical events that predisposes them to addictive behaviors. This can make it more difficult to adopt a healthful lifestyle, so it is crucial to identify this and address it to successfully change eating behaviors.

People with low self-esteem do not realize that they are living out a self-fulfilling prophecy. The belief that they are not worthy of attention makes it a reality. We are wired to operate in accordance with our beliefs, and it all happens outside of our awareness. A person who believes that he or she is unworthy will shy away from other people, develop habits that further lower their attractiveness to others, ultimately reinforcing their negative beliefs and practices. In doing so, such people often lower their self-perceived social status.

Status is an important factor that affects every facet of your life including the way that you eat. Although people think it has to do with class, economics, or education, it actually comes from something much deeper than that. It comes from a combination of what people believe about themselves and, most importantly for this discussion, what they believe others believe about them. In short, it is a measure of social acceptance. Lower-status people instinctively look to higher-status people for direction, without being aware of it. Lower-status individuals constantly seek acceptance through compliant behaviors, including eating, drinking, smoking and taking drugs.

Our self-esteem is a core belief; it deeply affects our behaviors in ways that we only barely perceive. Most of us are unable to judge our own status. To get an accurate measurement, we need to examine our automatic behaviors, the things we do without thinking. What are the principle indicators of low status and low self-esteem? A partial list of these includes:

- Conformity or compliance, especially with unhealthy behaviors; a fear of being different
- Social shyness or fear of displeasing others
- Lowered ability to communicate
- Involvement in dysfunctional family relationships
- Physical aggressiveness

We need to ask ourselves a series of questions to determine if we are allowing self-degradation to hurt our potential for healthful behaviors that will lead to success and happiness.

- Am I engaged in behaviors that are detrimental to me?
- What are the forces pressuring me to adopt or maintain this behavior?
- Does this behavior increase or diminish my status and self esteem?
- Am I a trendsetter or a trend-follower?
- Am I avoiding a useful behavior because I don't want others to think I am different?

We need to be able to view ourselves in a favorable light and cultivate behaviors and activities that build pride in ourselves in order to challenge these issues. That pride could come from helping others, being understanding of others, having interests that engage us, developing new skills, and appreciating value and goodness wherever we see it.

LIST A FEW REASONS YOU HAVE TO BE PROUD OF YOURSELF.

_____

_____

_____

_____

_____

_____

_____

_____

WRITE DOWN THREE THINGS YOU COULD DO TO EXPAND
THE WIDTH OR DEPTH OF YOUR INTERESTS.

_____

_____

_____

_____

_____

These written exercises may not seem to be directly tied to your desire to lose weight and increase your health. However, based on years of working with thousands of patients, I assure you that for many people they are. The key to change is learning social skills so you do not look for bad dietary habits to solve your social problems. Behaviors that lead to poor health lower your emotional well-being and further this cycle. Your beliefs and your diet work hand in hand. Self-confidence is important to your health and dietary choices. If you believe that what you say is worthwhile and attractive to others, this attitude will be transferred to everyone around you, regardless of how you might actually look. When you have a legitimate reason to believe in yourself, you will care for yourself better and be more inclined to eat right.

We are all prone to follow the direction of the group and most Americans follow a diet that is popular and unhealthy. Does following the crowd give you an excuse to resist change? It is a factor for some people. They want to fit in, and will be uncomfortable eating differently because they believe they will be rejected by their reference group. This perceived loss of status from being different can create a subconscious resistance, presenting another obstacle to change. This is an irrational response; following the crowd does not lead to enhanced status or self-respect. Quite the opposite; doing what you think is right will increase your self-esteem and emotional well-being. It is unfortunate that an unhealthy lifestyle and a disease-causing diet gains the psychological advantage as it certainly is more popular. But remember, you can lead the crowd; you can change things around for your social circle. By your example, you not only may save your own life, but you also may save someone else's life that you really care about.

Knowing that you have a group of friends, who help you to be a better person and with whom you have something in common, raises your emotional health and self-confidence. It is far easier to change and transition into a healthy lifestyle when you have the support of others doing the same. Look for support from people who will cheer you on. If they are not in your direct circle of friends or family, join a support group, locally or online. The more your group embraces and supports you in your efforts to eat better and live a health-supporting lifestyle, the easier this becomes. Our American reference group is a nation eating itself to death, committing suicide with their knives and forks. Given that, it is helpful to have support when attempting to move away from the dietary norm. If you have a real and tangible like-minded social group, you are much less likely to be affected by the artificial ones created by advertisers, marketers, and technology. If you want to get healthy, hang around other healthy people and others striving to be healthy.

Some people will attempt to make you uncomfortable because you are eating this way. Your change in behavior may make them uncomfortable because you are forcing them to examine their own practices. If you look for approval from someone who is struggling on that issue, you generally will not get a positive response. Don't let people with unhealthful and self-destructive food habits influence your food choices. Control your health destiny. Don't let the reaction of others subconsciously prevent you from adopting this program. Regardless of the illogical motives of the unconscious mind to save face, you actually lower your social status by letting these forces govern your choices.

Eating healthfully and developing the skills to earn and enjoy excellent health may increase your self-esteem, which in turn will help you socially. This is very important as we know from looking at the data on centenarians in Chapter 4.

The Australian Longitudinal Study of Aging showed that people with good relationships were 22 percent less likely to die over the following decade.[27] Interestingly, close contact with children and relatives had little impact on survival. It was those with the strongest network of friends and acquaintances who were the most likely to survive. Unquestionably, developing peers who are also interested in healthy living is a great idea. Forming a support group or even joining our online support group (www.DrFuhrman.com) can be extremely beneficial and aid in your success.

Knowledge Is Key
Even if you have fine self-esteem and a supportive group of people around you, your mind can hold you back from reaching the goals you have for your body. We most often behave in a manner consistent with the way we think. Some of the principles that you are learning as part of this eating-style may seem counter intuitive at first because they do not fit neatly into your prior beliefs. Because

we are social animals, ideas seem more believable when more people believe them. They require social proof before they gain general acceptance.

A study published in the *European Journal of Clinical Nutrition* looked at some of the factors that inhibit people from adopting a nutrient-dense, plant-based diet. The study found that the more knowledge subjects obtained about the benefits, the more they had their questions answered, and the more prior myths were shattered with science, the more likely they were to adapt to a healthy diet and achieve good health.[28] For some, change needs to occur in steps, and it has to be at their own pace. Remember, however, that your willingness to change and your success is proportional to the knowledge you obtain. This is a knowledge-based program. Gaining the knowledge is the most critical factor in facilitating behavioral changes that will lead to healthier habits.

Some will decide to ignore the life-enhancing information presented here. That decision is made on a subconscious level. A multitude of diets, nutritional supplements, and even drugs promise weight loss without changing the way you eat. These promises give the subconscious mind a way out, an excuse to do nothing, and often are enough to dissuade people from even considering change.

Many of these diets have been debunked, but that doesn't damage their allure to our subconscious minds where most decisions are made. The good news is that you are not at the mercy of your genes or your subconscious mind. You can control your health and weight. Heart disease, strokes, cancer, dementia, diabetes, allergies, arthritis, and other common illnesses are the result of incorrect dietary choices. With knowledge, you are empowered to make new choices.

Ideas have a life of their own. Once they are accepted and popular, they become difficult to displace. Much of what is now widely accepted as nutritional gospel is based on scant evidence, mistaken old notions, bad science, and myths advertised to us by food manu-facturers, pharmaceutical companies, and the government. These myths are so pervasive that even most scientists and physicians accept them.

Many current, popular dietary notions have uncertain origins, but since they have been around a long time, they generally go unquestioned. Once they become this ingrained, they are difficult to change and new information is hard to accept.

Here are some commonly held nutritional myths.

Frequent small meals aid weight control

FALSE—Frequent eating has been shown to increase calorie consumption. In addition, scientific studies, have shown that reduced meal frequency increases the life span of both rodents and monkeys, even when the calories consumed were the same in the group fed more frequently and in the group fed less frequently.[29] The body needs time between meals to finish digestion. Only when the digestion has ended, can the body most effectively detoxify and promote cellular repair. To maximize health, it is not favorable to be constantly eating and digesting food.

Being overweight is due to poor genetics

FALSE—Genetics do play a role in obesity, and people whose parents are obese have a tenfold increased risk of being obese. However, there are many people with obese parents who are slender and healthy. It is the combination of food choices, inactivity and genetics that determines the likelihood of obesity.[30] Excellent nutrition and a healthy lifestyle will overwhelm genetics and allow even those with a genetic hindrance to achieve a desirable weight.

Milk builds and strengthens bones

FALSE—Medical studies confirm that drinking cow's milk does not lead to stronger bones. In 2000, a comprehensive review of all studies on dairy intake and bone strength concluded, "the body of scientific evidence appears inadequate to support a recommendation for daily intake of dairy foods to promote bone health in the general population of the

United States."[31] First of all, vegetables are relatively high in calcium and when you eat healthfully you get plenty of it. However, having strong bones is about much more than just calcium. We require vigorous exercise, adequate vitamin D, and a healthful diet rich in many micronutrients. My nutritarian diet is ideally designed for bone health. It not only provides adequate calcium from vegetables but it is low in animal protein and salt, two dietary components that increase urinary calcium excretion, contributing to bone loss and osteoporosis. [32]

Heart disease and dementia are the consequence of aging

FALSE—Interestingly, heart disease as a major cause of disability and death is a recent phenomenon in human history. Heart disease has identifiable causes, and populations whose lifestyle practices do not create these causes do not have heart disease. Cultures around the world eating a nutrient-dense, vegetable-rich diet have no recorded heart disease, including hundreds of thousands of rural Chinese.[33] Diets that are high in animal fats and low in vitamins, minerals, fruits, and green vegetables, also have been shown to be related to the incidence of dementia.[34]

What criteria do you use for accepting new knowledge? Much of the information that I am presenting to you may be difficult to accept because it questions conventional wisdom and is based only on what can be proven with scientific evidence. Our cognitive models are based on our perceptions and feelings, not on actual facts. It is not the situation itself that determines what we feel, but rather it is the way we **think** about the situation. Learning this material might require you to change your way of thinking and, therefore, change your subconscious cognitive model. It will happen gradually and naturally as you go through the exercises and as your body changes as a result of your new eating patterns.

In the realm of health education and health care, misinformation abounds. Misinformation actually works hand in hand with self-deception. Countless diets advertise that you can eat all of the foods you love and still lose weight. Consequently, why would anyone want to completely revamp his or her diet? It seems like it would be far easier to eat less of something that you love than it would be to switch to eating something that you may not currently like. The problem is that, in practice, this has been proven not to work.

Studies have shown that portion control diets result in significant weight loss that is maintained over five years for fewer than three people out of 100.[35] These diets are doomed to fail because they do not satisfy our biological need for nutrients, and we continue to crave more calories than we actually require. In addition, these diets reinforce the low-nutrient eating that we now know causes most medical problems in modern countries. They are founded on weak science and perpetuate nutritional myths. To become healthy, disease-proof, and permanently thin, you can't escape the necessity of eating large amounts of nutrient-rich food.

Why We Believe Things That We Know Are Not True

If we were completely rational, all of our decisions would be based squarely on either facts or evidence. But, we are often not rational, and even people with a complete command of the facts will not make sound decisions.

Consider addicted smokers. They can tell you all of the reasons why smoking is harmful, yet for reasons they cannot articulate, they simultaneously believe they are better off continuing their addiction. Both their emotional and physical addictions prejudice their judgment, and they make rationalizations to believe something that clearly is not true.

Before we judge them, it should be noted that most Americans have heard over and over again that fruits and vegetables are the healthiest foods and are important to eat in larger amounts to protect against heart disease and cancer. Nevertheless, people typically dismiss or diminish the importance of this message. Their subconscious is not comfortable with change, and their subconscious wins. Inertia, the resistance of our ego to a change in its state of prior beliefs, prevails.

All of our actions and decisions are governed by our core beliefs. Our core beliefs define the limits of what we will and will not do. You may need to change your core beliefs in order to get healthy. At this point, you know that eating more vegetables has health benefits, but you may not really feel that this life-saving information will give you control of your health destiny, save you from suffering with pain, and add many quality years to your life. Your subconscious mind hasn't accepted it yet. For many people, the partial knowledge that they have acquired is in conflict with their core beliefs. They are unable to accept it, so their awareness of it dims and, with it, the ability to make the changes.

Psychologists have long observed that we all subconsciously dim awareness to things that raise our anxiety or make us uncomfortable. Our self-deceptions often lead us into absurd situations that are completely obvious to outside observers. Many people blame the media and big business for the current state of the American diet. The truth, however, is that Americans are self-deceived. There is nothing that prohibits us from choosing healthful foods, but contradictions often arise between the subconscious and rational portions of our minds. We are prone to believe what we want to, regardless of the evidence. Our brains are masters at suppressing facts.

Changing our ingrained habits requires that we operate for a period of time with cognitive dissonance. Cognitive dissonance is a psychological term describing the uncomfortable tension that may result from having conflicting thoughts, or from engaging in behavior that conflicts with one's beliefs. It usually results in the filtering of new information that conflicts with what one already believes. When it comes to choosing new eating habits and developing new taste preferences, cognitive dissonance needs to be recognized so we can get over it and move on. We must face the facts, accept our discomfort, and work through it.

Your subconscious might not be comfortable with the changes you are trying to make, but you have to hang in there until the change feels natural. Your taste preferences will change with time. The first step, of course, is getting started. In recognizing your discomfort, you will be able to acknowledge it and move on, so that you move one step closer to taking control of your health.

CHAPTER SEVEN

DEVELOPING A TASTE FOR HEALTH

Healthy Food Doesn't Taste Bad

Long established beliefs about health and food have created a cognitive model for our society, and that model affects your eating habits. One of the key principles you need to learn that goes counter to this cognitive model is taste subjectivity. Your tastes can be changed. We live in a food-obsessed society. Most people believe that their sense of taste represents something that is particularly unique to them. This is not the case; in recent years, our taste preferences have been hijacked and altered by manufacturers of artificial foods.

Consider the following statement: *"Healthy foods taste bad."*

Is that true? Inherently, no, but many people in our society would agree. If taste was something fixed and unchangeable, then this would create a problem for those people who want to eat healthfully. Being healthy would require us to eat things that do not taste good. Being healthy, therefore, would be an unnatural and illogical state. However, taste is not fixed. It is a learned response. The idea that a food "can grow on you" is true.

Our tastes are the result of our bodies adapting to the foods that we eat on a regular basis. Before the advent of refrigeration and global commerce, we could only eat foods that were grown locally.

Notice how people in different regions have different tastes. Are they born with different taste preferences than we are? No, their tastes have simply adapted to the foods in their region.

What does the phrase "healthy foods taste bad" really mean? By itself, the phrase means that people have adapted their taste preferences to prefer the unhealthy food they generally eat. However, what if they could change their preferences so that they would not only enjoy, but also prefer the taste of nutrient-dense foods? This can happen as you put this program to the test. Over time, as you practice eating these foods, you will begin to enjoy them more. As you complete the "Exercises with Food", sample new recipes, and slowly decrease your intake of processed and other empty-calorie foods, you will notice that your taste preferences will adapt. It's one of the many amazing changes that you will see by making this high nutrient diet an integral part of your lifestyle.

> *"We can't solve problems by using the same kind of thinking we used when we created them."*
>
> Albert Einstein

These words of wisdom from Einstein can be applied to your eating habits. The thought process that caused you to gain the excess weight will not be helpful as you try to lose it. You must be willing to let go of the old ideas that no longer serve you and never really did. Your health and weight are governed by the law of cause and effect.

Most people don't fail because of a lack of effort. The most common mistake that prevents people from achieving their goals is that they do the same thing over and over, illogically expecting a different result. They get locked into a single way of looking at things. Taking a different approach requires us to think differently. Here, it requires us to rethink what we consider a healthful diet. For a moment, consider the old definition of the standard grain-based diet and the tenets of my nutrient dense vegetable-based eating-style:

NUTRITARIAN DIET	STANDARD DIET
Vegetable-based	Grain-based
Lots of beans, nuts, and seeds	Lots of dairy and meats
At least three fresh fruits daily	Lots of refined sweeteners
Oils used sparingly	Oils used liberally
Animal products minimized (zero to four times a week)	Animal products emphasized (two to three times a day)
Focused on nutrient-dense calories	Focused on nutrient-poor calories

You can see that a major overhaul is required in your way of thinking to strive for a healthful diet. However with time and focus, eating the nutritarian way will become what tastes good to you.

Inflexible Palate Syndrome

This notion that food preferences can't be changed is so common that I have given it a name: inflexible palate syndrome. An inflexible palate is one that does not tolerate new foods. It prevents people from even starting to change their lives. People who have this syndrome believe that they can't eat better because they don't like the taste of healthful food. But remember, our tastes are subjective, learned responses to the foods that we eat on a regular basis. By systematically changing the foods that we eat, we can reprogram our perceived taste responses. By following the guidelines in this book, this syndrome can be eradicated. The menus and recipes I have included can be a tremendous help in this regard.

The inflexible palate syndrome is an impediment. An impediment blocks you from achieving a desired goal. There may be many impediments on your road to better health. Good health however, is governed by the law of cause and effect. When you start eating healthful whole foods, the desired effect will follow. The underlying habits required to achieve good health are all learnable skills.

Reprogram Yourself

As a society, we have programmed ourselves to eat in a way that is unnatural and harmful. We mistakenly prefer the taste of harmful foods. The most natural and healthy way of eating now seems strange, and eludes us. The benefits of eating natural foods, as opposed to processed foods, seem obvious, yet they are lost to many. Here are a few of the common excuses that I hear from people:

"It takes too much effort and time to prepare fresh food."

"I don't like the taste of fruits and vegetables"

"People will think I am strange if I eat this way."

Even if you don't voice these objections, you may still be thinking them. They form the core of your inner dialogue. This kind of talk is not useful. Its purpose is to prevent you from taking action. It is a type of learned helplessness; you don't believe you can succeed so you create a rationale for not trying. Right now, resolve to fight those thoughts when they enter your head. These excuses are not based on facts. They are opinions formed before adequate knowledge was available, and as you now know, knowledge is the cornerstone to success. Your internal programming and fixed beliefs can have you fail before you even start. This internal programming operates outside of your conscious awareness, yet it influences your thoughts and actions.

Psychologists tell us that both preconceived notions and the inner dialogue that resists change to preexisting beliefs are automatic thoughts. An automatic thought is an unconscious process that determines how we interpret the events of our lives. In many people, these thoughts are negative, pessimistic, and completely illogical. They persist because they operate beyond awareness and because they go completely unquestioned and unchallenged. Our automatic thoughts are the result of our core beliefs, and our core beliefs establish our perceived boundaries of what we can and cannot do.

The key to reprogramming yourself is to select an activity that elicits the desired objective, and then perform this activity habitually. As you continue to perform this activity, your skill will improve, your brain will reprogram to the preferred wiring, and your desired outcome will manifest itself. Your brain is not only flexible and adaptable, but it will restructure itself to accommodate whatever lifestyle you wish to create.

For years athletes have done visualization exercises to rehearse their physical specialties completely in their minds. They use their minds to train their bodies. Scientists have discovered how this works. In one study, subjects were instructed to raise their arms while their brains were scanned. They were then instructed to simply think about the act. The limbic brain patterns were identical. The athlete simply learns how to reproduce the same limbic pattern while she is performing it. Similarly, using PET (Photo-Emission Tomography) scan technology, neuroscientists have observed that people with similar lifestyles and circumstances have similarly structured brains.

Consider taxi-cab drivers in London. London streets are very complex. Taxi drivers go through extensive training and are required to know the best route and alternates between any two addresses. When the brains of these taxi drivers were scanned, researchers discovered that they all had unusually large hippocampus regions. The hippocampus is the part of the brain used to handle spatial orientation and navigation. What was even more interesting was that the size of the hippocampus was proportional to the time that the individual had driven the cab. The activity or skill of being able to drive a cab through a complex maze like London caused the hippocampus to continuously grow, long after the period of active study ended.[36] For both athletes and these taxi drivers, practicing their skills changed their brains. For you, practicing how you want to eat will change how your brain works in relation to your food preferences.

Just as you cannot expect to develop a perfect tennis swing or learn how to play a musical instrument without both good instruction and a tremendous amount of practice, you cannot hope to transform your health without the ongoing process of putting your new knowledge into action. Moving in the right direction, improving the way you eat, and learning how to handle social situations that encourage bad habits are all part of an ongoing process of change. It is a process that requires time and effort and the ability to learn from mistakes. As the saying goes, practice makes perfect. It is not enough simply to know what to do. You need to do it. You need to practice preparing recipes and eating super-healthful meals until such time as they begin to satisfy your desire for pleasurable eating.

Anyone who has become accomplished at demanding activities, such as sports and music, will tell you that it can be difficult to learn new things. It is not easy to develop new habits, and there is no such thing as a shortcut to developing new skills and expertise. Likewise, it takes practice and perseverance to eat healthfully.

When you do something over and over, it creates a pathway in the brain that makes it easier and more comfortable to repeat it again later. That is one reason why it is so hard to change a person with ingrained bad habits. For example, I would rather teach someone who never played tennis before how to properly swing a racket than to try to teach someone who has been playing for years and swings incorrectly. That's why teaching this high-nutrient eating-style to children from an early age is such a good idea. They don't have the bad habits ingrained, so it is easier to accept. However, while change may be difficult, it is not impossible. What is needed is a strong desire and motivation to change, a willingness to be uncomfortable, and a determination to work on it until you get it right.

The more you make healthful meals, and the more days you link together eating nutrient-dense foods, the more your brain will naturally prefer to eat this way. Your taste for healthful foods will develop. It has been shown that a new food needs to be eaten about fifteen times for it to become a preferred food. The more days you eat healthfully, the more you will lose your addiction to unhealthful, stimulating substances. With time, you will look forward to—and prefer eating—a diet that is more natural and wholesome.

Your Diet, Your Choice

One day, I asked myself why I eat the way I do. What is my motivation? What do I get out of it? So what if I die younger? Why not just enjoy all the processed food our high-tech, modern world has to offer? Why not eat cheeseburgers, fries, soda, and ice cream for lunch, and take my chances with an earlier death? At least I will enjoy the time I am alive, right?

In thinking about it, I realized that I actually enjoy being a nutritarian and eating this way. I believe I get more pleasure from eating than people who live on unhealthy food because I've learned to appreciate the tastes and flavors of natural foods, and I know I'm doing something good for myself. I would eat this way anyway, even if there was a slight decrease in the pleasure of eating, but after years of eating like this, I prefer it. The fact that it is good for me is certainly the largest attraction, but health-destroying foods are not appealing to me anymore. However, I have complete freedom to eat anything I want, and if I occasionally want to eat something unhealthful, I do. But, over the years, I have found that I desire unhealthful foods less and less because I do not feel well after eating them. Plus the taste is not as pleasurable as I anticipate it will be.

There are great tasting, high-nutrient alternatives to tempting but unhealthful foods. These alternatives make it easier to choose to eat right. I do not feel deprived. So, I eat the way I am advocating you eat. I am not overweight and I am not on a diet. I may not eat perfectly all the time, but I have balanced pleasure and health in my diet so that I am not sacrificing one to have the other. I eat this way for a lot of reasons:

- I enjoy this way of eating. It tastes great, and I like to eat lots of food.

- I want control of my health and want complete assurance I will not suddenly have a heart attack or stroke.

- I enjoy living too much. I love sports, travel, entertainment, exercise, my work, and my family, and I want to maintain my youthful vigor and enjoyment of life.

- I feel well eating this way and do not like the way I feel, the way I sleep, my digestion, or my mental energy when I do not eat this way.

- I want to live longer and without medical interference, pain, and unnecessary suffering in my later years.

Eating healthfully is an option, a choice. You have the right to care for yourself as you choose. Others may choose to continue to engage in risky behaviors, using the rationale that a pleasure-seeking, life-shortening option is preferable. The fallacy is that people who smoke, drink, take drugs or eat dangerous foods are enjoying life more. In fact, they enjoy it less because the harmful results of their addictive behaviors remain long after the temporary pleasure has vanished.

Toxic habits and disease-causing foods actually inhibit your ability to get pleasure from eating. A healthier body means stronger taste buds. Your taste buds become less sensitive from chronic excess exposure to sweets, salt, and other harmful substances. Food then tastes bland. You lose the ability to appreciate the subtle variety of flavors in natural foods, and you become dependent on using excess sugar and salt.

Eat healthfully, and over time you will prefer eating healthfully. Delicious, even gourmet recipes can be designed for a high-nutrient diet. It is almost insane to commit suicide with a disease-causing diet.

People who have adopted my nutritarian advice have reversed long-standing conditions, including autoimmune diseases, diabetes, headaches, and heart disease and have been brought back from the brink of death. All this simply by changing the way they eat. Sadly, a very large number of people are simply unable to even attempt this change. Their habits now control them, and they are no longer in total control of their lives. I urge you—don't be one of them.

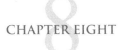

CHAPTER EIGHT

EXERCISES WITH FOOD: THE WORK OUT

Now that you have warmed up to healthful, high-nutrient whole foods, it is time to turn the workout routine up a notch. I want you to start eating so many more vegetables and fruits that they become the foundation of your diet.

In this work out, we will focus on palate stretching exercises. Instead of stretching your biceps with barbells, you will be stretching your palate and digestive system with a variety of raw and conservatively cooked, natural foods.

It's okay if you don't love the taste of these foods at first. When you eat a meal, you expect to like what you are eating. However, when you are exercising it is okay not to like the exercise while you are doing it because you are not exercising for its own sake. You are looking forward to the increase in muscle or endurance that comes afterwards. When trying a new healthful but unfamiliar dish, you might not enjoy the taste at first. You might even think you will never enjoy it. More likely, you just need to give your taste buds a little time to get used to it.

We can call this exercise "eating without taste expectations". Going through this phase is a necessary step for people who want to achieve great health. It is helpful while doing the palate stretching to concentrate on the physical benefits of the foods that you are eating. Habitually stretching your palate will increase your exposure to healthy foods until over time, you will prefer their tastes.

EXERCISE 3

Take the half-pound of vegetables and half-pound of fruit that you are eating daily and increase them to one pound each per day. The pound of vegetables can be raw or cooked. Eating two salads daily—one of vegetables and one of fruit or whatever combination you feel like—is not too much. To help you meet your vegetable goal, eat a bowl of vegetable bean soup or a vegetable bean casserole each day. The recipes at the end of this book can help you along the way. Don't forget to try some of my delicious salad dressing recipes with your salads and raw vegetables.

EXERCISE 4

While you add more volume to your diet, also change the types of fruits and vegetables that you are eating. Alternate at least three different fruits and three different vegetables in your diet each week. Also, I encourage you as part of this exercise to try a fruit or vegetable that you rarely eat or have never tried. This is a good opportunity to see the palate stretching in action as you realize that your tastes can change. Grocery stores today have plentiful produce departments that most likely contain something you've not yet discovered. Be adventurous. Stretch your palate and your experience in an effort to have a more complete diet.

WORK OUT GOALS

1. Eat one pound of fruit and one pound of vegetables daily. The pound of vegetables can be a combination of raw and cooked.

2. Eat a bowl of vegetable bean soup or a vegetable bean casserole or stew daily. You can try my recipes or select no-salt-added or low sodium varieties from the store.

3. Use my delicious salad dressing recipes with your salads and raw vegetables.

4. Alternate at least three different fruits and three different vegetables in your diet each week. Experiment with new fruits and vegetables.

There Will Be Roadblocks

As we have discussed, there are many impediments on the road to becoming truly healthy. For many people, they can include having low self-esteem, lacking a support group, feeling hesitant about giving up foods, and not wanting to take the time to gain the knowledge necessary for change. Place a score of 1 to 10 on the lines below to indicate the strength of that obstacle in your life:

_____ I don't know if I can learn to like the taste of nutrient-dense foods.

_____ I don't know if I can give up unhealthful foods that I like.

_____ I don't know if my family will eat these foods.

_____ I don't want to eat differently from other people.

_____ I don't know if my friends and relatives will like me eating this way.

_____ I don't know how I will eat in business, traveling, and social situations.

_____I don't know if I can manage the time to
prepare foods like this.

_____ I don't know if I can find enough time to
exercise regularly.

_____I don't know if I can make the time to shop
for food.

_____I don't know if I can learn to cook
healthful food.

_____I don't like to cook.

_____I can't afford to spend more money on food
than I do now.

_____I hear so much conflicting information about
nutrition, I don't know what's true.

_____Diets never worked for me in the past, so I
would rather not try.

_____I can't lose weight no matter what I do.

_____Other roadblock _____

_____

People can always come up with an excuse why something is too difficult to do. The subconscious mind is great at this, but a strong desire and commitment on your part to achieve your wellness and weight goals can silence these objections. With planning and support, you can reduce the intensity of each of the roadblocks, and eventually eliminate them.

Re-visit this page over the course of following this plan, both when you are feeling comfortable and when you are encountering difficulties. When you are hitting a rough patch, remind yourself that you are in control. You have consciously evaluated the difficulties, and while that doesn't remove them, it should stop you from using them as a crutch. When you revisit this page during a comfortable time, score these roadblocks again. You will see the number of roadblocks decrease, indicating how gaining the knowledge and living the plan is changing your thought process.

CHAPTER NINE

THE COMPLEXITIES OF HUNGER

"When I started following Dr. Fuhrman's plan after reading *Eat To Live*, I learned about the ideas of being addicted to food and feeling the desire to eat too frequently and too much. As I read the description of addiction, I realized that was me exactly. After eating a bagel and yogurt every morning, I could not make it to lunch. I had to have more coffee and some chocolate as a pick-me-up in between meals, otherwise I would develop a mild headache and feel listless. At lunch, a light salad would not do it.

I needed the heavy, cheesy dressing to feel fulfilled and normal. I realize now that I was in a vicious cycle of feeling low unless I ate regularly and kept my blood sugar up. It was tough to break the addictions at the beginning, but I followed the plan and made it through until my body didn't feel dependent upon those foods anymore. Now I feel nothing between meals. I feel fine when my blood sugar is low, and I don't even feel like eating then. It is so much more pleasurable to eat when I am really hungry, instead of being driven by my food addictions.

Eight months after beginning the program, I am 60 pounds lighter and still losing, but I am no longer dieting to lose weight. I am content eating pleasurably and healthfully because I feel so much better. In fact, for the first time in years, I actually have the energy to exercise!

Eating this way has also had an effect on my family. My husband changed his way of eating. At first, it was just to support me, but then he began to notice that his eyesight was improving. As he continued to follow the plan, he was able to lower his eyeglass prescription, go off of the cholesterol-lowering drugs that he had been on, and lose 40 pounds. With both of us eating this way, our kids are slimmer, healthier, and learning valuable lessons about food for the rest of their lives."

Robin Rossi
Glendale, Arizona

Moving Forward

Like Robin and her husband, if you continue to follow the instructions in this book, you will see remarkable physical changes as a result of the increasing health your body is experiencing. Depending on your current age and state of health, you will witness a transformation as the pounds melt away and your biological clock is literally turned back. You will be able to physically see that a high-nutrient, lower-calorie diet actively restores and preserves health and a youthful appearance, while a diet low in nutrients and full of empty calories accelerates aging.

At this point on your road to great health, we focus even more on nutrients. For the remainder of the book, when I refer to nutrients, I will be referring specifically to micronutrients, not macronutrients. As we continue to replace low-nutrient items with foods of high nutrient density, remember there are foods that you can eat in unlimited quantities (assuming no overeating) because they have extremely high levels of nutrients per calorie. They are:

- All fresh fruit

- All beans and legumes

- All vegetables, except potatoes

In the menus at the end of this book, you will find that the amount of animal products is limited, and most of the oil in your salad dressings will be replaced with avocados and nuts, which are full of important nutrients. With oil, even olive oil, the hidden calories can add up fast, sabotaging your weight loss. Since all oil is 120 calories per tablespoon, it is a substance you want to use in minimal amounts. When you do choose to use oil on your salad or in your cooking, use only a teaspoon per person. It is part of the process of gradually reducing calories from low-nutrient foods and replacing them with calories that have higher nutrient values.

The Four Dimensions of Hunger

We commonly call the feeling of wanting or needing to eat "hunger," but to understand hunger, we need to address four important considerations: volume, nutrients, calories and addictions. Many diets fail because they only focus on one of these components—calories. *Eat For Health*, based on the ideas developed in *Eat To Live*, is the only eating-style that takes into account all four.

1) VOLUME—You must consume an adequate amount of food, and fiber from that food, to physically feel satiated.

2) NUTRIENTS—You must consume enough nutrients in your food for your body to meet its biological need to thrive. Even if you have adequate volume, if it's from low-nutrient food, your body will have a nutrient deficit, and you will feel the need to eat more food.

3) CALORIES—You will be driven to overconsume calories unless you get enough volume and nutrients for your body to feel satiated.

4) ADDICTIONS—You must put an end to your addictions to food, which often manifest themselves in discomfort and cravings. If you don't, your body will not be able to regulate its caloric needs appropriately.

As you can see, each of these dimensions addresses your body's need for food, but none of them exists independently. If one dimension is not tended to, the others will be thrown off. Portion-control diets attempt to limit calories without regard to nutrients or volume. Hunger is never fully satisfied and the undernourished dieter ends up giving in to the overwhelming compulsion to eat more. We have discussed the importance of nutrients and calories and how the two work together. Now we will address the main reason that people eat too much and become overweight: food addiction.

Emotional Addictions

Lots of people are overweight, and most of them know being overweight is not good for their health. Often, their friends and family and even their doctors have advised them to lose weight, but they can't. They have tried various diets and simply can't stick with them.

People often overeat for emotional comfort. It can bring fleeting pleasure. Food can be a drug-like outlet to dull the pain and dissatisfaction of life, but like drug or alcohol use, it is never a good long-term solution. It only winds up complicating things further. What people of all body weights really want is to feel proud of themselves. This cannot be achieved by overeating and eating unhealthily. Packing on additional pounds leads to more guilt and self-hate and, subsequently, more overeating to dull the pain. The solution to this cycle must include more than just food menus and diet plans; an emotional overhaul is needed.

Your eating for comfort has to be replaced with other outlets that build self-esteem and offer solace in emotionally healthy ways. For many people, these outlets can include feeling proud of yourself for exercising, for kindness to others, for doing a job well, for developing a new skill, and for making more choices that will improve your future health. Losing weight can be a powerful boost to your self-confidence and self-esteem. In other words, the more reasons you have to feel good about yourself, the increased likelihood you will succeed in every aspect of your life. Your new attitude must be one that lets go of the idea that you are stuck with your lot in life and that you can't change things. You can. When you are overweight and you lose weight, you can see it, as can everyone around you. It is a visible representation that you have changed and you have taken back control of your life.

Once you experience how effectively the high-nutrient diet can transform your health, drop excess weight, and dramatically heighten your emotional well-being, you will stop coming up with rationalizations why the effort is not worth it. However, to realize those rewards, you first must put this program into action. Getting healthy takes considerable focus and effort. You need to plan and put time into this. Of course, it is easier to eat processed and convenience foods and claim you are too busy to squeeze exercise into your schedule, but the effort to do what it takes is well worth it. It will allow you to transform your health and set you free to enjoy a much more pleasurable life. When you make the commitment to take proper care of yourself and put out the effort, you take back control.

These emotional issues are tied into the act of eating for many people, so there is no need to feel alone in experiencing them. If you are someone who experiences these issues, it is helpful to have a friend or a social support so you can share and discuss these topics. It is crucial to address them while also addressing the strong physical addictions that almost every person eating the standard, toxic, American diet has developed.

Food Addiction Starts the Fat Cycle

Almost every person eating the standard, toxic American diet develops strong physical addictions. It is crucial to address and resolve these addictions. When a heavy coffee drinker stops drinking coffee, he feels ill, experiencing headaches and weakness, and even feels nervous and shaky. Fortunately, these symptoms resolve slowly over four to six days. Discomfort after stopping an addictive substance is called withdrawal, and it is significant because it represents detoxification, or a biochemical healing that is accomplished after the substance is withdrawn. It is nearly impossible to cleanse the body of a harmful substance without experiencing the discomfort of withdrawal. Humans have a tendency to want to avoid discomfort. They continue their toxic habits to avoid unpleasant withdrawal symptoms. When we discontinue consuming healthy substances, such as broccoli or spinach, we do not experience discomfort. We feel nothing. Only unhealthful, toxic substances are addicting, and, therefore, these are the only substances that cause discomfort when you stop consuming them. Their addictive potential is proportional to their toxicity.

Uncomfortable sensations are very often the signals that repair is under way and the removal of toxins is occurring. Though it may be difficult to adjust to this way of thinking, feeling ill temporarily can be seen as a sign that you are getting well. That cup of coffee may make you feel better temporarily, but any stimulating substance that makes you feel better quickly, or gives you immediate energy, is hurtful, not healthful. Any substance that has that immediate effect is toxic and called a stimulant. Healthy foods do not induce stimulation. When you meet your needs for nutrients and sleep, your body will naturally feel well and fully energized, without the need for stimulation.

The more you search for fast, temporary relief with a candy bar, a can of soda, or a bag of chips, the more you inhibit the healing, detoxification process. Your body becomes increasingly toxic as you give it more low-nutrient calories. Calories consumed without the accompanying nutrients that aid in their assimilation and metabolism lead to a build-up of toxic substances in the cells that promote cellular aging and disease. Eating low-nutrient calories increases dangerous free-radical activity within the cells and allows for the build-up of cellular waste. These low-nutrient calories also increase other toxic materials in the body, such as Advanced Glycation End Products (AGEs). AGEs affect nearly every type of cell and molecule in the body, and are major factors in aging and age-related chronic diseases. Their production is markedly accelerated in diabetics, and they are believed to play a causative role in the vascular complications of the disease.

AGEs are the result of a chain of chemical reactions and may be formed externally to the body by overcooking foods or inside the body though cellular metabolism. They form at a constant but slow rate in the normal body and accumulate with time, but their formation can be accelerated by your eating habits. The secret to aging more slowly and remaining youthful is to prevent the accumulation of AGE's in the body.

Dry cooking methods such as baking, roasting, and broiling cause sugars to combine with proteins to form AGEs, while water-based cooking, such as steaming and boiling, does not. AGEs are high in burnt and browned foods, and overcooked animal products, but these compounds also can build up in cells from the consumption of low-nutrient calories, especially calories from sweets. So, eating both overcooked foods and low-nutrient foods leads to the build-up of AGEs and ages us faster. When you eat a diet that is based on toxic and addictive foods—such as salt, fried foods, snack foods, and sugary drinks—you not only build up free radicals and AGEs in your cells, but you also set the stage for feeling ill when you are not digesting food. Unhealthy food causes your body to create waste by-products that must be removed by the liver and other organs. Only when digestion ends can the body fully take advantage of the opportunity to remove toxins. If the body is constantly digesting, it can't go through this detoxification process effectively.

When detoxification begins, people often feel queasiness or malaise. Eating something restarts digestion and shuts down the detoxification process, making the bad feelings go away. The lower the nutritional quality of your diet, the worse you will feel if you try to stop eating food for a few hours. You will only feel normal while your digestive tract is busy.

Toxic Hunger

After years of eating a poor diet, detoxifying your body can be both physically and psychologically difficult. The latter is involved because people often think that, since eating makes them feel better, the symptoms of detoxification are actually hunger. This leads to one continuous eating binge all day. It is no wonder that 80 percent of Americans are overweight. Every few hours they are compelled to put something in their mouths. They may feel better temporarily from that chocolate-chip cookie or pretzel, but they never really get rid of the uncomfortable symptoms. The symptoms come back again and again.

I call these detoxification (withdrawal) symptoms toxic hunger. It will recur whenever digestion ceases, not when the individual is truly hungry and has a biological need for calories. Toxic hunger keeps coming back to haunt you every time your digestive apparatus is no longer busy digesting. Because you feel the desire to eat so frequently, you will become overweight, and, in the process, your opportunity for a long life and disease-free future is lost.

Food addiction affects almost all Americans. It takes superior nutrition to lose the symptoms of toxic hunger. Toxic hunger makes it almost impossible to reduce portion sizes, cut back on calories, count points or follow other typical dieting strategies. You can't easily stop overeating when you are a food addict. A person can't be expected to eat less food when they feel so bad when they do. Unless people are informed, they mistake the withdrawal symptoms they feel for hunger, or claim they have hypoglycemia and they simply can't help eating too frequently and too much. Once you address your addictions and use this knowledge to help yourself through the detoxification process, you will be able to more easily, efficiently and pleasurably address your nutrient and caloric requirements.

Toxic hunger is a physical addiction to an unhealthful, low-micronutrient diet. Its symptoms are generally feelings that we have been taught to interpret as hunger. However, they are actually signs of your body's toxicity.

SYMPTOMS OF TOXIC HUNGER

- Headaches

- Weakness, shakiness and fatigue

- Stomach cramping

- Light-headedness

- Esophageal spasms

- Growling stomach

- Irritability and inability to concentrate

These uncomfortable symptoms are experienced to different degrees by different individuals. Sugary foods with a high glycemic index can fuel these symptoms and the toxic hunger eating frenzy, but consuming too many animal products can do it too. Americans are now accustomed to eating animal products, including beef, chicken, eggs, and cheese, at every meal, but eating such a high quantity of these very high protein foods can overload the liver's ability to eliminate excessive nitrogenous wastes. The excessive consumption of animal proteins and the elevated amount of waste products puts a stress on your body's detoxification channels and you wind up not feeling well—or detoxifying more—between meals.

Some people are more sensitive to this excess nitrogen than others. It is not unusual to find people who are forced to eat a diet rich in protein and animal products. Otherwise, they feel too ill. They must remain on a continual high-protein binge all day. They feel terrible if they try to stop eating high-protein foods or if they delay eating. These individuals may feel better when eating animal products at regularly spaced intervals, but this is the same as drinking more coffee to feel better.

It leads to more and more addictive symptoms and they never get better. Just like the caffeine addict, they may have to feel worse for a short time for these symptoms to resolve. Even though the overeating of animal protein causes the problem, the high-protein food also temporarily allows them to feel better and to feel better longer after the meal because high-protein foods take longer to digest and can delay the discomfort of withdrawal.

Eating again to remove those uncomfortable feelings never gets you off the overeating merry-go-round. You can have another cup of coffee or slice of cheese in an attempt to feel better, but it is this cycle that caused you to become overweight and suffer these ill feelings in the first place. To get rid of the toxic hunger symptoms that drive overeating behavior, you may have to feel uncomfortable for a few days to resolve the issue. I frequently have people make a gradual change in their diet to minimize the discomfort. Eventually as they are able to change the diet more and more, they lose the hypoglycemic symptoms and are able to feel comfortable delaying eating or eating less. This is a necessary first step for them to get back in control of their overeating. Toxic hunger is the main reason people fail on diets. Toxic hunger is a primary cause of obesity in the modern world. We have adopted a toxic diet, and because of it, we are forced to overeat.

True Hunger Can Help You Be Healthy
My high nutrient diet can set you free from your food addictions and allow you to lose your toxic hunger. The food cravings will end

and you will be able to stop overeating. Then, you will be back in contact with true hunger. When you achieve that, you will be able to accurately sense the calories you need to maintain your health and lean body.

I want to reiterate that as you adopt a high-nutrient eating-style, it is common to go through an adjustment period in which you experience fatigue, weakness, light-headedness, headaches, gas, and other mild symptoms. This generally lasts less than a week. Don't panic or buy into the myth that to get relief you need more heavy or stimulating foods, such as high-protein foods, sweets, or coffee.

The feelings associated with these symptoms are not how true hunger feels. It is our unhealthy tendency to eat without experiencing true hunger that has caused us to become overweight in the first place. To have become overweight, a person's food cravings, recreational eating, and other addictive drives have come into play. Poor nutrition causes these cravings, and superior nutrition helps normalize or remove them. You will no longer need to overeat when you eat healthfully.

True hunger is not felt in the stomach or the head. When you eat healthfully and don't overeat, you eventually are able to sense true hunger and accurately assess your caloric needs. Once your body attains a certain level of better health, you will begin to feel the difference between true hunger and just eating due to desire, boredom, stress, or withdrawal symptoms. The best way to understand true hunger is to experience it for yourself. It has three primary characteristics:

❶ A SENSATION IN YOUR THROAT

❷ INCREASED SALIVATION

❸ A DRAMATICALLY-HEIGHTENED TASTE SENSATION

Being in touch with true hunger will help you reach your ideal weight, and you also will feel fine whether you eat, delay eating or skip a meal. Almost all of my patients who suffered with headaches and so-called "hypoglycemia" have gotten well permanently following my nutritional recommendations.

How True Hunger Works

People generally snack between meals to satisfy toxic hunger and food cravings, or they consume empty calories and toxic food for recreational purposes. Recreational eating is eating because you are in a social setting or simply because there is food around you. Recreational eating can still occur without satisfying toxic hunger or true hunger. Sometimes people— including me—just enjoy eating good-tasting food when it is offered, even though we are not feeling any symptoms directing us to eat. When most people eat in this way, they do it with junk food, not healthful, natural foods. The way we can reduce recreational eating is by experiencing how much more enjoyable it is to eat when we are really hungry. Then we find that the food tastes much better. This heightened taste sensation that accompanies true hunger gives us terrific feedback to inhibit overeating behavior so we can actually get more pleasure out of our diet. Delaying eating, to the point when true hunger is experienced, makes even ordinary foods taste great and extraordinary foods taste even better.

In our present toxic food environment, we have lost the ability to connect with the body signals that tell us how much food we actually need. We have become slaves to withdrawal symptoms and eat all day long when there is no biological need for calories. This is not in harmony with our natural physiology. In an environment of healthful food choices, we do not feel any signals to eat until hormonal and neurological messengers indicate that glycogen reserves in the liver are decreased and lean body mass will soon be used as an energy source. Our bodies have the beautifully orchestrated ability to tell us exactly how much to eat to maintain an ideal weight for our long-term health. These signals are what I call true hunger. This name also differentiates it from toxic hunger, which is what everyone else, refers to simply as hunger. Most Americans have not felt true hunger since they were toddlers.

Feeding yourself to satisfy true hunger cannot cause weight gain. If you only ate when truly hungry, it would be almost impossible to become overweight. True hunger is a signal to eat to maintain your muscle mass. Eating to satisfy true hunger does not put fat on your body. Excessive fat stores are developed only from eating outside of your body's true hunger demands. When you get back in touch with true hunger, you will instinctually know how much to eat. When you exercise more, you will get more and more frequent hunger; when you exercise less, you will get much less hunger. Your body will become a precise calorie-measuring computer and steer you in the right direction just from eating the amount that feels right and makes food taste best.

True hunger is not uncomfortable. It does not involve your stomach fluttering or cramping. When you feel it, you know it is a normal reaction that signals a need for food. It signals that the body is physiologically ready to digest, and the digestive glands have regained their capacity to secrete enzymes appropriately. It makes food taste much better when you eat, and it makes eating much more pleasurable. People are consistently amazed at how good the simplest foods can taste when they are truly hungry.

I have observed this changing perception of hunger in thousands of individuals who adopted my high-nutrient diet. I have documented this discovery in scientific studies and explained the biochemistry behind it. It is a fundamental principle of this diet-style and it can free you from the prison of addictive overeating.

True hunger requires no special food to satisfy it. It is satisfied by eating almost anything. You can't crave some particular food and call it hunger. A craving by definition is an addictive drive, not something felt by a person who is not an addict. Remember, almost all Americans are addicted to their toxic habits. A disease-causing diet is addicting. A health-supporting diet is not.

To consume the exact number of calories necessary to maintain a lean body mass that will prolong life, you must get rid of toxic hunger and get back in touch with true hunger. If you eat only when hungry, you will never have to diet or be overweight again. You do not have to carry around a calculator and a scale to figure out how much to eat. A healthy body will give you the correct signals. You will only desire the amount of calories you actually require.

Getting Enough Volume

Our hunger drive craves volume. A key skill that you are developing is the ability to eat large volumes of raw and cooked, high-nutrient, low-calorie foods every single day. This means eating lots of vegetables. It may be helpful to look again at the image of three stomachs from Chapter 5. Each is filled with the same amount of calories, but one in the form of oil, one in the form of chicken, and one in the form of vegetables. The stomachs with the oil and chicken have a great deal of room in them, room that can enable you to easily overeat on calories. That's why filling your stomach with high-nutrient foods is so important to achieving and maintaining a healthy weight. This leads us to a counter intuitive, but crucial rule: to lose more weight, and for better health, eat more high-volume, low calorie foods. To lose more, eat more.

When you are actively trying to lose weight, you should strive to satisfy your volume requirements first, before addressing the other components of hunger. This may feel strange at first because you may not immediately feel satisfied by the higher volume of food. This is because you are accustomed to eating large quantities of high-calorie foods that cause a dopamine rush, a rush that low calorie foods don't deliver. However, your body will adjust, be less dependent on the dopamine surge in the brain, and will gradually become more and more satisfied with fewer calories. Give yourself time, and use the knowledge you have gained. Striving to fulfill your body's volume and nutrient requirements can help you resolve your food cravings and your toxic hunger.

The trick to get you to desire fewer calories faster is to eat a lot of these high-volume, high-nutrient foods. You are already familiar with these, since many of the foods that you have been incorporating into your diet because of their nutrient values are also great tools in meeting your volume requirements. They include:

RAW VEGETABLES—lettuce, tomatoes, peppers, celery, snow pea pods, carrots, beets, cucumbers, red cabbage, onion, bean sprouts

FRESH FRUITS—berries, melons, oranges, pears, apples, grapes, kiwis, peaches, papaya, mango, cherries

COOKED GREEN VEGETABLES—kale, collards, Swiss chard, brussels sprouts, spinach, string beans, artichokes, asparagus, broccoli, Chinese cabbage, bok choy, zucchini

COOKED NON-GREEN VEGETABLES— mushrooms, eggplant, onions, cauliflower, spaghetti squash, butternut squash, carrots

On holidays and other times when you know that you will be around a lot of unhealthy foods, fill up with these high-nutrient, low-calorie foods. Never go to a party or event with an empty stomach. Eat a large salad with assorted raw vegetables and a bowl of vegetable soup before going to the places that may tempt your desire to eat unhealthfully. Being healthy is about being in control. You must control your hunger, and the more low-calorie, high-volume foods you consume, the less high-calorie food you will be able to eat. When you increase these super-healthy foods in your diet, you will feel less temptation, and you will be in control of your food cravings and appetite.

CHAPTER TEN

UNDERSTANDING YOUR ADDICTIONS

More than two-thirds of Americans are overweight. This is to be expected. People should expect to become overweight when they do not meet their needs for nutrients and volume. It turns them into food addicts, and they are forced to overeat on calories. Processed foods, low-nutrient eating, and high-protein diets based on animal products create food addictions and derail true hunger.

Understanding and managing your hunger is a critical key to creating the physical environment that will help support your efforts to earn longevity and superior health. The body's drive to feed itself is part of the design to maintain optimal health, which includes ideal weight. It is geared toward self-preservation and its purpose is to make the body thrive. The irony is that people seem to have appetites bent on self-destruction. These are unnatural appetites.

Our ability to enjoy unhealthy foods is the result of an otherwise useful ability to adapt to a variety of environments. This was useful in the past when food was scarce. Processed and unhealthy choices were unavailable. Our tastes were designed to enable us to enjoy whatever food we could obtain from the natural environment. It helped us to distinguish foods from poisons. In today's toxic food environment, the survival drive for calories can direct us to the most calorie-concentrated processed foods. Our innate drive for calories has been shackled by the food manufacturers peddling white flour, salt, sweeteners, and artificial flavors. The more you eat low-nutrient, processed foods, the more you crave these substances. It is almost impossible not to over-consume calories and gain weight when your diet is so low in nutrients.

Dangers of Salt

Salt consumption is linked to high blood pressure, blood clots, heart attacks, and stomach cancer. You might be thinking, "Wait a minute. I have low blood pressure. Why do I have to worry about salt?" The answer is that even if you have low blood pressure now, 90 percent of all Americans eventually develop high blood pressure from their high sodium intake earlier in life. Once it is high, it is not so simple to bring it down again with the removal of salt. Instead, you wind up on medication to lower it.

Raised blood pressure is a major cause of death in the world and, in most countries, 80 percent of the adult population is at risk.[37] High blood pressure is mostly the result of a poor diet, lack of exercise, and excessive salt consumption, but according to the Journal of the American College of Cardiology, salt consumption is a significantly bigger risk factor than the other elements.[38] If you already have high blood pressure, eating a low-salt, whole-food diet can remedy your condition and potentially save your life. Even if your blood pressure does not come down with the removal of salt, do not think salt doesn't matter for you. It may take a long time for your body to undo the damage from the many years of excessive salt intake. For those people who have normal blood pressure, removing salt from your diet and following the proper dietary recommendations will mean you won't have to worry about taking medications later in life and you will get more protection against stroke and heart attacks than medications can offer.

High sodium intake is predictive of increased death from heart attacks. A recent study of adults with pre-hypertension showed that over the ten to fifteen years that the individuals lowered their sodium intake by at least 25 percent, their risk of cardiovascular disease correspondingly fell 25 percent. The conclusion is that consuming a high amount of sodium will put you at greater risk for heart disease and shortened life.[39] In another recent study, high sodium intake was predictive of coronary heart disease and mortality from heart attacks, independent of other risk factors, including blood pressure. This means that it is not just about raising blood pressure. More and more direct evidence is emerging that salt is harmful to the heart in other ways.[40] Salt also causes calcium and other trace minerals to be leached from your body, which is a contributory cause of osteoporosis. As excess salt is removed via the urine, other minerals such as calcium and magnesium accompany it and are lost as well.

I understand that as you follow this high-nutrient plan, increasing your intake of fruits and vegetables and decreasing your intake of animal products and saturated fats, you may be tempted to ignore the salt factor. You may say, "I'm already making these big changes. I can't deal with taking salt away as well." However, there is another very important reason why we are gradually reducing salt intake. Studies have shown that a certain type of stroke, called a hemorrhagic stroke, increases as heart attacks decrease in a population.

As the consumption of animal products, saturated fat, and processed foods drops down to low levels in a population's diet, heart disease goes to lower and lower levels, reaching less than one percent of the total causes of death. Eating a diet lower in saturated fat and higher in fruits and vegetables dramatically reduces the occurrence of the clots that cause heart disease and embolic strokes.

However, hemorrhagic strokes are not caused by atherosclerosis—the buildup of fatty substances in arteries—and the resultant clots. These strokes are caused by a hemorrhage or rupture in a blood vessel wall that has been weakened by years of elevated blood pressure as a result of chronic high salt intake. The weakened wall ruptures and lets blood flow into and damage brain tissue.

Although whole food vegetarian and flexitarian diets that include the occasional or minimal use of animal products may markedly reduce the risk for coronary heart disease, diabetes, and many common cancers, the real Achilles heel of no-animal-fat and low-animal-fat diets is this increased risk of hemorrhagic stroke at an older age. This is because animal products and processed foods contribute to plaque formation called atherosclerosis. Atherosclerosis promotes blood clots that cause heart attacks and embolic strokes. However, this process may also thicken, and therefore protect, the small, fragile blood vessels in the brain from rupturing due to the stress from chronic high blood pressure. When a diet is high in fatty animal products and processed foods, the thickened blood vessel walls caused by the unhealthful, heart-attack-promoting diet actually protect against the occurrence of this more uncommon cause of strokes. In medical studies, higher cholesterol levels are associated with increased risk of other strokes, but lower risk of hemorrhagic strokes.[41]

Admittedly, these types of strokes cause a small percentage of deaths in modern countries, but that is because so many people die prematurely of heart disease or cancer that they don't live long enough to experience this additional detrimental effect of their high-salt diets. However, for those striving to maximize their lifespan, it is even more important to avoid a high-salt intake.

Decreasing Salt, Increasing Taste

Now that you understand why salt must be dramatically lowered in your diet, you may still be questioning how you will do it without eating bland food every day. Part of the answer is that you won't be entirely eliminating sodium. To do that is impossible because all foods, especially vegetables, contain sodium, and this natural sodium adds to their flavor.

Up until now, you have probably never noticed this natural sodium. When our taste buds are over-stimulated with too much added salt over a long period of time, our taste receptors can't sense lower levels of salt. Natural, unsalted foods seem to have less flavor.

Food tastes flat without added salt, and you need to add more salt to almost everything. This is part of the addiction cycle; we build up tolerance for unhealthy substances. The good news, however, is that you can retrain your taste buds to be more sensitive to salt when you decrease its presence in your diet.

Most people consume between 2000 and 8000 milligrams of salt each day. When you get rid of the salt habit, your food may taste bland for a few weeks, but you will find that your taste buds, which were deadened by the overuse of salt, gradually regain their sensitivity. You will discover tastes that you never knew existed in natural foods. Even a simple pear or a leaf of lettuce tastes better. Foods that you previously enjoyed will taste too salty.

When you eat a diet low in salt, eventually your sensitivity to salt and other tastes gets stronger. As you eventually get accustomed to a diet that stimulates your salt-receptive taste buds less, you can enjoy more flavors in natural foods. This stronger taste ability isn't just limited to the taste sensation of salt. You also will see the phenomenon at work when eating a simple strawberry or slice of red pepper. Amazingly, your taste buds become stronger when you are off salt and sugar. Try eating some plain romaine lettuce with no dressing on it now. Then eat some after reducing your salt intake and following my high-nutrient program for a month. You will be amazed at how much more flavor that plain, unseasoned piece of lettuce has.

The bottom line is that once you break your addiction to salt, you won't miss it at all, and you will find that food actually has more flavor not less. High-nutrient eating strengthens your senses as it improves your health.

Limiting Saturated Fat

Autopsy studies on adult Americans who die in car accidents, unrelated to heart conditions, demonstrate that heart disease is present in the vast majority of American adults. Almost all people over the age of 40 are found to have a significant amount of atherosclerosis in their coronary arteries.[42] The bottom line is, if you eat the Standard American Diet or something close to it, you most likely will develop the same diseases—heart disease, high blood pressure, stroke, dementia, and cancer—that most Americans get. You cannot escape from the biological law of cause and effect. Our long-term health is determined by our food choices.

We get heart-healthy fats in their natural, high-antioxidant environment when we eat raw seeds and nuts. Indeed, avocado, nuts, and seeds are rich in fat. They may even contain a small amount of saturated fat, but their consumption is linked to substantial protection against heart disease. Unfortunately, in the American diet, fats come primarily from meat and dairy, which are saturated, and we compound the problem by the low level of food-derived antioxidants and phytochemicals we ingest.

Saturated fat comes from many food sources, including processed foods, meat, cheese, and other animal products. Thousands of scientific research studies demonstrate that saturated fat promotes both heart disease and cancer and powerfully raises cholesterol.[43] However, the avoidance of all fat is not the secret to protecting your heart. The secret is avoiding saturated fat, trans fats and processed oils.[44] These fats do not contain the fat-binding sterols, phytonutrients and antioxidants present in high-fat, whole plant foods. When people eat high-glycemic processed foods along with animal fats and low-nutrient oils, it leads to cardiovascular disease, depresses the immune system and increases the risk of cancer.[45]

The table on the following page shows the saturated fat in some common foods. Small amounts of saturated fat are not dangerous, but remember, you should be striving to eat much less saturated fat compared to most other Americans. You will see it is possible for people to ingest thirty or even fifty grams of saturated fat each day without thinking too much about it. Comparatively, a healthful diet typically contains less than five grams of saturated fat.

SATURATED FAT CONTENT OF COMMON FOODS[46]

	Grams of Saturated Fat		Grams of Saturated Fat
Cheddar cheese (4 oz)	24	Chicken thigh no skin (6 oz)	5
American processed cheese (4 oz)	24	Whole milk 3.3% fat (one cup)	5
Ricotta cheese (one cup)	20	Plain yogurt	5
Swiss cheese (4 oz)	20	Two eggs	4
Chocolate candy semisweet (4 oz)	20	Chicken breast (6 oz)	3
Cheeseburger large double patty	18	Salmon (6 oz)	3
T-bone steak (6 oz)	18	Walnuts (2 oz or 24 halves)	3
Braised Lamb (6 oz)	16	2% Milk (one cup)	3
Pork –shoulder (6 oz)	14.5	Tuna (6 oz)	2.6
Butter (2 tbsp)	14	Turkey, white, no skin, (6 oz)	2
Mozzarella, part skim (4 oz)	12	Almonds 2 oz (48 nuts)	2
Ricotta cheese part skim (one cup)	12	Sunflower seeds (2 oz)	2
Beef-ground-lean (6 oz)	11	Flounder (6 oz)	0.6
Ice cream, Vanilla (one cup)	10	Sole (6 oz)	0.6
Chicken fillet sandwich	9	Fruits	negligible
		Vegetables	negligible
		Beans/Legumes	negligible

While consuming high amounts of saturated fat is clearly dangerous, it is not the only villain. Keep in mind that consuming fats that raise your cholesterol is only one of many factors that increase your risk of heart disease, strokes, and dementia. Excessive blood cholesterol is also the result of eating a low-nutrient diet that causes increased free radicals and heightened intravascular inflammation. This inflammation results in increased cholesterol production and deposition of atherosclerotic plaque. High fiber, natural plant food on the other hand, binds cholesterol in the digestive tract and removes it. Therefore, your cholesterol level goes up when you don't eat enough vegetables and beans. Saturated fat, and especially trans fat, causes higher cholesterol levels than simply eating cholesterol does. For example, eggs are high in cholesterol, but eating eggs will not raise your cholesterol as much as eating cheese because cheese is much higher in saturated fat.

Studies in the United States and Europe have established that the incidence of death by coronary heart disease is nearly two-and-a-half times higher for people with the highest 25 percent of blood cholesterol, compared with people with the lowest 25 percent. Yet the coronary heart disease mortality for the same cholesterol levels is only one-third as great in Japan and the Mediterranean.[47] In other words, a person in Scotland with the same blood cholesterol levels as a person in Catalonia, Spain, is eight times more likely to die of coronary heart disease. It is the higher intake of fruits and vegetables in the Mediterranean area that makes the difference.

LDL cholesterol, or bad cholesterol, is the one we want to watch. LDL is very fragile and susceptible to oxidization, which means the fat is partially rotten due to a build up of free radicals. This oxidization is a critical factor in the depositing of plaque on blood vessel walls.[47] Fruits, vegetables, beans, seeds, and nuts are our primary source of antioxidants. Consuming enough of these foods can reduce the negative effects of LDL oxidization. Again, the problem is not just saturated fat. It is this interaction between saturated fat and the low nutrient environment that makes it a more powerful villain.

A recent study looked at the effects of a diet with more fruits and vegetables combined with a low saturated fat intake. It showed a 76 percent reduction in heart-disease-related deaths for those consuming more than five servings of fruits and vegetables per day and less than 12 percent of calories from saturated fat, compared to those with less vegetation and more saturated fat.[49] Even this small increase in vegetation and mild reduction in saturated fats showed a dramatic reduction in heart-disease-related deaths. Can you imagine the heart protection that would be possible with 10 servings of fruits and vegetables and less than five percent of calories from saturated fat? You simply do not have to develop, suffer from, and die of heart disease if you achieve superior nutrition.

Complicating the issue here regarding saturated fat is that animal foods, even the ones low in fat, are high in protein. High intake of animal protein raises blood levels of insulin-like growth factor one (IGF-1), which heightens one's risk of cancer and accelerates aging.[50] Foods that may be low in fat, such as egg whites and white meat chicken, still promote cancer since they so effectively raise IGF-1. The other confusing issue is that when studies evaluate people who consume less fat and more refined carbohydrates such as sweets, bread and pasta, they do not see a reduction in heart disease deaths because the negative effects of refined carbohydrates are just as bad as high saturated fat intake. Some have interpreted these findings to give them the license to eat more high-fat animal products. The fact that poorly designed low-fat diets are still atherogenic (causing the formation of plaque in the inner lining of arteries), in no way minimizes the risk of eating a diet rich in fats and animal products. We must recognize that both of those dietary factors are disease-promoting. By contrast, when your diet is predominantly unrefined plant foods, rich in greens, beans, seeds and nuts and you are free from the negative effects of refined carbohydrates, saturated fat and animal protein, you optimize longevity.

The Worst Meat Options

Red meat and processed meats contain more saturated fat and trans fat than other animal products, and are the poorest food choices. However, the fat issue does not tell the whole story. Scientific studies have documented that red meat has a much more pronounced association with colon cancer and pancreatic cancer compared with other animal products.[51] The consumption of red meat and processed meats on a regular basis more than doubles the risk of some cancers. Even ingesting a small amount of red meat, such as two to three ounces a day, has been shown to significantly increase the risk of cancer.[52]

Toxic nitrogenous compounds (called N-nitroso compounds) occur in larger concentrations in red meat and processed meats. Red meat also has high haem (also spelled heme) content. Haem is an iron-carrying protein, and it has been shown to have destructive effects on the cells lining our digestive tract.[53] Processed meat, luncheon meat, barbecued meat, and red meat must not be a regular part of your diet if you are looking to maintain excellent health into your later years of life.

Eating too many animal products and not enough vegetables increases one's risk of cancer. To achieve optimal health, humans require a high exposure to a full symphony of phytochemicals found in unprocessed plant matter. Eating more animal products results in a smaller percentage of calories consumed from high phytochemical vegetation such as seeds, berries, vegetables and beans. Also, since animal products contain no fiber, they remain in the digestive tract longer, slowing digestive transit time and allowing heightened exposure to toxic compounds.

You should reduce your consumption of animal products gradually until you're only consuming them two to three times per week. Of course, I recommend totally avoiding processed meat and barbecued meat.

Fish Is Not a Health Food

Many people believe they are improving their diets by eating less meat and more fish. Since fish is generally low in fat and high in beneficial omega-3 fats, many consider it an important part of a healthy diet. Studies have demonstrated that when people eat less red meat and more fish, health outcomes are improved. However, a review of the literature on fish consumption shows that fish is a double-edged sword because it may also contain mercury and other pollutants.

In spite of the presence of valuable omega-3 fats, called EPA and DHA, nearly all fish and shellfish contain mercury and other pollutants, such as PCB's. Pollutants and mercury accumulate in fish as the polluted water is filtered through their gills. Larger fish that have lived longer have the highest levels of mercury because they've had more time to accumulate it. They may also accumulate it from all the smaller fish they have eaten, similar to the way we accumulate mercury in our tissues from the fish we eat.

If you eat fish regularly, your body is undoubtedly high in mercury. You cannot remove the mercury by trimming the fat or by cooking because it is deposited throughout the fish's tissues. Mercury levels tested in patients correlate exceptionally well with the amount of fish the individuals consumed.

Individuals eating fish a few times a week had blood mercury levels exceeding 5.0 micrograms, the maximum level recommended by the National Academy of Sciences. Women eating seafood more than twice per week had seven times the blood mercury levels of non-fish eaters, and children eating fish regularly had mercury levels 40 times higher than the national mean.[54] Mercury can be removed from the body naturally, but, even after a patient avoids fish for a period of time, it may take years for the levels to drop significantly.

The bottom line on fish is we can no longer consider it a health food. Either avoid it or eat it no more than once weekly. If you do have fish, chose from the lower-fat, lowest mercury types, such as flounder, scallops, trout, sole, squid or salmon.

Avoid swordfish, mackerel, tilefish and shark. They contain the highest mercury levels.[55] Be aware of the place where it was caught and what type of fish it is. Never accept recreational fish from questionable waters, and never eat high-mercury-content fish. It is not worth the risk.

If the consumption of toxins from fish has potential health risks, wouldn't it be better to get our omega-3 fats from a cleaner source? Yes. It is safer to rely on a clean, low-dose, DHA-EPA supplement, such as my DHA-EPA Purity (www.DrFuhrman.com), or a clean fish-oil supplement taken a few times a week instead of eating potentially contaminated fish. Since my DHA-EPA Purity supplement is not fish-derived, you are assured of achieving adequate DHA and EPA levels without mercury and other pollutants. When buying these omega-3 supplements, keep in mind that they should be purchased from a well-documented, reliably clean source, close to the date of manufacturing, and refrigerated upon receipt.

Detriments of Dairy

The consumption of cheese has skyrocketed in recent history. Dairy is the food category that contributes the most saturated fat to the American diet, and cheese and butter are now the major contributors. As you can see from the saturated fat chart, compared with the same size piece of fowl or fish, cheese could have ten times as much saturated fat. However, the high saturated fat content of dairy is not the primary reason to limit its consumption.

Cow's milk is the perfect food for a rapidly growing calf. There is a clear association between high-growth-promoting foods such as dairy products and cancer. There is ample evidence implicating dairy consumption as a causative factor in both prostate and ovarian cancer.[56] Dairy protein boosts the amount of insulin-like growth factor (IGF-1) in the blood. IGF-1 is found in cow's milk and has been shown to occur in increased levels in the blood of individuals consuming dairy products on a regular basis. IGF-1 is know to stimulate the growth of both normal and cancer cells. Case control studies in diverse populations have shown a strong and consistent association between IGF-1 concentrations and prostate cancer risk.[57]

The link between lactose (milk sugar) and ovarian cancer was investigated as part of the Nurses' Health Study, which enrolled over 80,000 women. Researchers reported that women who consumed the highest amount of lactose (one or more servings of dairy per day) had a 44 percent greater risk for all types of invasive ovarian cancer than those who ate the lowest amount (three or fewer servings monthly). Skim and low-fat milk were the largest contributors to lactose consumption.[58]

Given this clear link between increased consumption of even low-fat diary and skim milk and cancer, it is wise to reconsider dairy as an important source of calcium in the diet. This is another reason why animal source foods should be limited. When you eat sufficiently from whole plant foods, you get plenty of calcium.

Nutritarian Diet vs. Vegetarian Diet

As you know by now, the foundation of the nutritarian diet is the dramatically increased consumption of micronutrient-rich vegetables, fruits, beans, seeds and nuts. Vegans (vegetarians who consume no animal products) and vegetarians (who consume dairy products and/or other products obtained from animals) can take advantage of the high-nutrient diet as long as they follow all of the protocols. Typical vegetarian and vegan diets do not include such a large amount of high-nutrient, whole plant foods, and therefore do not offer as much in terms of improved health or longevity. Vegans and vegetarians who consume a largely plant-based diet will get some of the advantages of the high-nutrient diet, but the benefits do not come primarily from the abstinence from animal products. The benefits come from eating more vegetables, beans, fruit, nuts and seeds compared with those eating more conventionally.

Vegans and vegetarians whose diets center around processed cereals, white flour products, rice, white potato and processed soy products should not expect to significantly extend their life span because their diets cannot be considered nutrient-rich. The reduction in consumption of animal products is only one important feature in the design of an optimal diet, not the focal point. The critical issue for disease reduction is the nutrients-per-calorie ratio of a given diet. Unfortunately, in addition to large amounts of processed foods, vegan and vegetarian diets typically contain high amounts of added salt, which is extremely unhealthful.

You do not have to exclude all animal products from your diet to follow this plan and receive profound benefits to the health of your blood vessels and the rest of your body. You just have to reduce them to safe levels, as demonstrated in the menus and recipes included in this book.

Humans are primates, and all other primates eat a diet of predominantly natural vegetarian. While the great apes occasionally eat smaller animals, it is a very small percentage of their total caloric intake. Likewise, modern medical studies confirm that for humans to maximize their potential for a long, disease-free life, they have to keep animal product consumption to a relatively small percentage as well. Animal products are low in micronutrients, contain almost no antioxidants and phytochemicals, and are high in calories. They should be limited if you want to thrive in your later years, not just survive long enough to reproduce and then deteriorate.

In the standard American diet (SAD), less than 5 percent of the total caloric intake comes from nutrient-rich foods. This dangerously low intake of unrefined plant foods guarantees a weakened immunity from disease, leading to frequent illnesses and a shorter life span. When you eat a truly health-supporting diet, you can expect not only a drop in blood pressure and cholesterol and a reversal of heart disease, but also the elimination of headaches, constipation, indigestion and bad breath. Achieving this means eating fewer animal products and less processed food, sugar and flour, and eating more high-nutrient plant foods and exercising. This lifestyle shift is the key to disease protection in general.

Processed Food Dangers

Trans fats are extremely dangerous to the body chemistry. Trans fats are man-made fats that are used in processed foods. They are modified vegetable-derived fats that may be even worse than animal-derived saturated fats. They are also called hydrogenated oils, and they are laboratory-designed to have a similar chemical structure as saturated fat. They are solid at room temperature and have adverse health consequences. Like saturated fats, they promote heart disease and cancer.

When you are reading food labels and you see the words "partially hydrogenated" on the box, it is another way of saying trans fat, so avoid it. If you avoid processed food, it is easy to avoid trans fat.

In addition to trans fats, the baking of grains and potatoes causes browning of the food and the formation of a hard crust, which is rich in acrylamides. Researchers have found that many of the processed foods we eat contain these cancer-causing compounds. Acrylamides form in foods that are browned by being fried, baked, roasted, grilled, or barbecued, but not in those that are steamed, boiled or sautéed in water. Water-based cooking prevents the browning or burning that forms these harmful compounds. Frying and overcooking lead to the highest levels of acrylamides, the highest of which are found in processed cheeses, fast food meats, fried chips such as potato chips, french fries and sugar-coated breakfast cereals.

Even though these chemicals have been shown to be potent carcinogens in animal models, so many acrylamides are consumed in the modern world that good research documenting the extent of the cancer risk in humans does not yet exist. This topic is still being actively investigated in many different countries, but the risk is difficult to estimate because baked, browned, and fried foods are so ubiquitous in Western diets.

European governments permit far less acrylamides in packaged foods than the U.S. and, they have been advising food manufacturers to reduce them. Cereals and processed foods manufactured in the United States are not under such restraints and have much higher acrylamide levels. Since the same browned and hard-baked products are also rich sources of the Advanced Glycation End Products previously discussed, there are plenty of reasons to minimize or avoid these foods in your diet.

The Caffeine Drug

As you know, caffeine is one of the most addictive substances in a standard diet, and there is some research that indicates that excessive consumption of caffeinated beverages may pose a risk to your well-being. Coffee, however, does contain chlorogenic acid, a phenol with strong antioxidant activity which may benefit people who eat very few vegetables. So, in spite of hundreds of studies showing slightly increased risk of certain diseases such as osteoporosis and heart disease, there are also studies that show certain health benefits from coffee.[59]

Either way, both the risks and the supposed benefits are marginal. One or two cups of coffee per day are not likely to cause significant disease risks. An obvious problem with caffeine is that it is a stimulant, so it gives you the false sensation that you can comfortably get by on less sleep, and inadequate sleep promotes disease and premature aging.[60] Overall, it is difficult to discern the precise risks from heavy coffee drinking because most people who drink a lot of coffee participate in other unhealthy behaviors as well. Another perplexing variable in studies on coffee is that coffee drinkers generally don't drink as much soda, which is a lot worse than coffee, so that it can make coffee drinking seem beneficial.

My main objection to drinking coffee is that it is addicting and, therefore, may promote more frequent eating and a higher calorie intake in some people. Eliminating your caffeine intake may help you lose weight. Coffee drinkers—and tea and cola drinkers—are drawn to eat more frequently then necessary. They eat extra meals and snacks because they mistake unpleasant caffeine withdrawal symptoms with hunger. They can't tell the difference between true hunger and the discomfort that accompanies caffeine withdrawal.

In essence, coffee is mostly like a drug, not a food. In spite of the presence of some beneficial antioxidants, it also has some negative effects and withdrawal symptoms that may fuel drinking and eating. The polyphenols it contains could have some minor benefits, but its toxic effects and resultant risks likely overwhelm those minor advantages. It is best if we aim to meet our nutritional needs with as little exposure to stimulating substances as possible. This program will work more effectively if you are able to gradually reduce and eventually eliminate coffee and other caffeine-containing substances, so that you become better connected to your body's true hunger signals.

Giving detoxification a chance

It takes time to be comfortable with the changes in your life. In the process of making over your body chemistry with a healthful diet, it is not unusual to feel physically uncomfortable as you detoxify. The more stimulating or harmful your prior habits, the worse you feel when you stop them. When breaking your addiction to salt, meat, dairy, saturated fat, processed foods and other substances, you might feel headachy, fatigued, or even a little itchy or ill, but the good news is these symptoms rarely last longer than a week or two.

Some people are so addicted to stimulating food, sugary sweets, and overeating, they may even feel depressed when they don't indulge. For example, cheese, salt, and chocolate are all addictive, and it takes a prolonged period of abstinence to beat these addictions. Sugar and caffeine, especially when mixed together, are highly addictive and create a significant amount of discomfort when eliminated from the diet. Sugar withdrawal symptoms have been demonstrated to be similar to withdrawal symptoms from opiates, including anxiety and tremors.[61] I have observed many individuals with a history of severe chronic headaches, who were on drugs for headache suppression, develop fever, backaches, diarrhea, and other severe detoxification symptoms when stopping medications that contain caffeine, such as Excedrin, Fiorinal and Fioricet. Fortunately, their suffering was short-lived. Through high-nutrient eating, these individuals have been able to make dramatic recoveries.

High-nutrient eating is crucial for recovery from chronic headaches or migraines. Toxic wastes build up in our tissues, and we are unable to remove them unless high-levels of phytochemicals are present and the intake of toxins is stopped. These plant-based phytochemicals are necessary to enable the body's detoxification machinery. Before recovery can happen and before you can really feel your best, you must allow this detoxification to occur. An important hurdle to achieving your ideal weight and excellent health is getting rid of your addictions. After that occurs, you may feel like you have been freed from prison and will find it easier to move forward with this program. You will be one step closer to truly eating for health.

Once you learn how to prefer the most healthful foods, managing your hunger boils down to structuring your eating so you consume the maximum nutrition in the fewest calories. If you consume adequate volume and nutrients, the calories will take care of themselves. The nerves lining the digestive tract send signals up to the brain, which regulates eating behavior. When our nutrient and volume needs are unfulfilled, we desire more calories to feel satisfied, and we create food addictions.

When you eat with a focus on maximizing micronutrients in relation to calories, your body function will optimize, chronic illnesses such as high blood pressure, diabetes, and high cholesterol will melt away, and you will maintain your youthful vigor into old age. You may be surprised to find that excess weight drops off at a relatively fast rate, without even trying to diet or eat less. A consistent, ideal weight is easy to maintain when nutrient needs are met with a dietary program rich in vegetables, beans, and fresh fruits.

You simply don't want to overeat anymore. It's as if you had your stomach stapled, because once the micronutrient needs are met, it becomes difficult to overeat.

CHAPTER ELEVEN

HIGH-NUTRIENT FOOD CATEGORIES

Learn to Love Salads

Hundreds of population studies show that raw vegetable consumption offers strong protection against cancer.[62] The National Cancer Institute recently reported on over 300 different studies that all showed the same basic information: If consumed in large enough quantities, vegetables and fruits protect against all types of cancers, and raw vegetables have the most powerful anticancer properties of all foods.[63]

Sadly, fewer than one in 100 Americans consumes enough calories from raw vegetables to ensure this defense. I encourage my patients to eat two salads each day (or one salad plus a green smoothie or glass of freshly squeezed vegetable juice). To help you remember the importance of raw vegetables, put a big sign on your refrigerator that says, **"The Salad is the Main Dish."**

The word salad here means any vegetable eaten raw or uncooked. Fresh fruit, unsulfured dried fruits, beans, and a delicious dressing can be added to it. Eating a huge, delicious salad is the secret to successful weight control and a long healthy life.

This health-makeover program encourages you to eat raw vegetables in relatively unlimited quantities, so think big. Since they have a negative caloric effect, the more you eat, the more weight you will lose. A negative calorie effect means that the food contributes so few calories and is so bulky that it displaces space in the stomach, leading to a full feeling, which has the effect of limiting the consumption of other, more calorie-rich options. The high levels of micronutrients and fiber also help to control appetite. Typically, you eat fewer calories at meals that feature lots of high-nutrient and calorie-negative foods. Some foods, especially raw green vegetables, supply fewer calories (even if you filled your stomach with them) than the total number of calories needed for their digestion and other important metabolic processes prior to eating again. This means that you can eat large-sized portions of these foods and still lose weight because your body will need to burn its excess fat to meet basic metabolic needs.

Raw foods also have a faster transit time through the digestive tract, resulting in more weight loss than their cooked counterparts. The objective is to eat as many raw vegetables as possible (without overeating), with the goal of one-pound daily. An easy way to accomplish this is to eat a salad at the beginning of your lunch, and then have some raw vegetables with dip before dinner. This could be an entire head of lettuce with one or two tomatoes and some shredded peppers, beets, or carrots. Or, you could have cucumber and shredded cabbage with shredded apples and raisins, or raw broccoli, cherry tomatoes, and snow pea pods with a delicious humus or salsa dip. The possibilities are endless, and my menus and recipes detail many ways for you to deliciously reach this goal.

Though it may seem daunting, it is far from impossible to consume one pound of raw vegetables, especially if it is split between two meals. Believe it or not, an entire pound is less than 100 calories of food.

My long-time advice to eat a large amount of raw vegetables (a large salad) before lunch and dinner has been tested by the medical community. Researchers used a crossover design to track the calories consumed by the same people when they ate salads as an additional first course at a meal and when they didn't. The research showed that consuming salads reduces meal-calorie intake and is an effective strategy for weight control.[64] Raw vegetables are not only for weight control; they also promote superior health in general.

When you add one of my delicious fruit, nut, or avocado-based dressings to the salad, the monounsaturated fats in the dressing increase the body's ability to absorb the anti-cancer compounds in the raw vegetables.[65] The synergistic combination of the raw vegetables and the healthy dressing makes the salad a health food superhero.

Greens Are King

As we've discussed, all foods get their calories from fat, carbohydrate, or protein. Green vegetables, unlike high-starch vegetables like potatoes, get the majority of their calories from protein. When more of your protein needs are met from green vegetables, you get the benefit of ingesting a huge amount of critical, life-extending micronutrients.

The biggest animals all eat large amounts of green vegetation, gaining their size from the protein found there. Obviously, greens pack a powerful, nutrient-dense punch. Monkeys and apes are basically plant eaters. The greatest percentage of their daily diet comes from plant foods; they eat only small to negligible amounts of animal matter. These primates are estimated to take 95-99 percent of their diet exclusively from plant foods. The desire of these animals for a variety of plant foods in their diet supports nutrient diversity and enables them to live long lives, free of chronic diseases. The micronutrients that fuel the primate immune system are found in nature's cupboard-the garden and forest.

Humans are primates, too, and we have a very similar biology and physiology to other primates. Based on genetic information, chimpanzee and human DNA only differs by 1.6 percent. Without an adequate amount of plant-derived nutrients, we do not thrive. Our immune systems are compromised, and we develop frequent infections, allergies, autoimmune disease, and often cancer.

Low in calories and high in life-extending nutrients, green foods are your secret weapon to achieve incredible health. Scientific research has shown a strong positive association between the consumption of green vegetables and a reduction of all the leading causes of death in humans.[66] Cruciferous vegetables in particular, broccoli, Brussels sprouts, cabbage, kale, bok choy, collards, watercress, and arugula, to name a few, are loaded with disease-protecting micronutrients and powerful compounds that promote detoxification and prevent cancer.

HELPFUL HINT:

The cruciferous vegetables include kale, bok choy, cabbage, cauliflower, broccoli, broccoli rabe, broccoli sprouts, brussel sprouts, mustard greens, watercress, turnip greens, collards, arugula and radishes.

Since cruciferous vegetables are your best weapons against cancer, include plenty of them in your diet.

The recipes in this book include numerous cruciferous vegetable soups and stews. Eat a good portion of these vegetables every day.

To bring your body to a phenomenal level of health, my goal is to deliver these foods to your plate in a variety of ways that make them delicious and increase your absorption of their beneficial nutrients. Greens can be served raw in salads, steamed and chopped as part of dinner, and cooked in soups.

When we steam or boil vegetables some of the phytochemicals, vitamins, and minerals get lost in the water, but when we simmer vegetables in soup, all the nutrients are retained in the liquid. Additionally, the liquid base of the soup prevents the formation of toxic compounds that are created as food is browned under dry heat. Many beneficial chemical compounds are more readily absorbed when the food has been softened with heat.[67] If you have been looking through the many recipes and menus included at the end of this book, you have found that we incorporate larger quantities of greens in an assortment of delicious ways as you move up the stages of dietary excellence.

Frozen vegetables are also a convenient option. They are picked ripe and flash-frozen right on the farm, so they are rich in micronutrients. It is fine to substitute frozen vegetables in any of the recipes to cut down on your cooking time.

Starchy vegetables include winter squashes, corn, potatoes, cooked carrots, sweet potatoes, yams and pumpkins. Since they are more calorically dense than the non-starchy vegetables, they are limited to one serving daily for those who need to lose weight. White potato is not a high-nutrient food, and many studies reveal an association between a diet high in white potato and obesity and diabetes.[68] These studies may be biased by the way potatoes are consumed (often fried or loaded with butter or sour cream), but, nevertheless, because of their relatively low nutrient density and their high glycemic index they should play a minor role in your diet. Sweet potatoes, carrots, and peas are much healthier options.

It is convenient to place whole grains, such as brown and wild rice, quinoa, millet, and whole wheat in this starchy category too, but keep in mind that the colorful, high-starch vegetables such as carrots and sweet potato and black or wild rice are higher in nutrients compared to most of the grains. Whole grains are wholesome foods, but should play a smaller role in the diet as Americans eat too many grains and not enough vegetables and beans.

Fresh Fruits Fight Cancer

Fresh fruits are an important component of the natural diet of all primates. Humans and other primates have color vision and the ability to appreciate sweets. We are designed this way so that we can recognize ripe fruits and be attracted to them. We have a natural sweet tooth designed to direct us to those foods most critical for our survival.

Sugar and candy manufacturers also know that bright colors and sweet tastes are instinctually attractive. They have used that knowledge to their advantage. Remember, your instinctual reaction is designed to lead you to fruit—not sugary, processed foods. Fruit is an indispensable requirement to maintain a high level of health. Fruit consumption has been shown to offer the strongest protection against certain cancers, especially oral, esophageal, lung, prostate, and pancreatic cancer.[69]

Researchers also have discovered substances in fruit that have unique effects on preventing aging and deterioration of the brain. Some fruits, particularly berries, are rich in phytochemicals that have anti-aging effects. Studies have shown that blueberries have protective effects for brain health in later life.[70] In addition, certain pectins—natural parts of the cellular makeup of fruits such as oranges, kiwis, and pomegranates—also lower cholesterol and protect against cardiovascular disease.[71]

As you can see, fruit is vital to your health and well-being and can contribute to lengthening your life. I use fresh and frozen fruits to make delicious desserts that are healthy and taste great. Many delicious and easy fruit recipes are provided in the recipe section of this book to satisfy your sweet tooth. When you complete your evening meal with one of those recipes—a frozen strawberry sorbet, a cantaloupe slush, or simply a bowl of fresh berries—you are putting the finishing touches on a meal that will satisfy your desire for a sweet food, while intellectually satisfying your desire to be healthy and wise.

You should always keep a good supply of fresh fruit on hand. It is the ultimate "convenience" food. Try to eat a variety of fruits: apples, apricots, bananas, blueberries, cherries, clementines, dates, figs, grapes, kiwis, kumquats, mangoes, melons, nectarines, oranges, papayas, peaches, pears, persimmons, pineapples, plums, pomegranates, raspberries, strawberries, and tangerines. Try some exotic fruits to add variety and interest to your diet.

If you are diabetic or on an aggressive weight loss plan, eat more fruits that are lower in sugar such as berries, green or Granny Smith apples, melons, oranges, kiwis and papaya and less of the higher calorie fruits such as mangos, grapes, bananas, pineapple and peaches. Those with diabetes do not need to avoid fruit as long as they limit it to two fresh fruits with breakfast and one with lunch and dinner. They should exclude fruit juice and eat only limited amounts of dried fruit.

Frozen fruit can be a convenient substitute when fresh fruit isn't available. The nutritional value of frozen fruit is comparable to that of fresh fruit. Avoid the canned varieties because they are not as nutritious. They often have sweeteners added and they have lost most of their water-soluble nutrients.

Beans or Legumes

Beans are among the world's most perfect foods. They stabilize blood sugar, blunt your desire for sweets and prevent afternoon cravings. Beans contain both insoluble fiber and soluble fiber and are very high in resistant starch. Although resistant starch is technically a starch, it acts more like fiber and "resists" digestion. Since it passes through the small intestine undigested, it means that a significant amount of the carbohydrate calories are not absorbed. Therefore, beans can make you feel full without adding all of their calories to your waistline.

Bean intake recurs in scientific studies as an important factor promoting long life. The conclusions of an important longitudinal study show that a higher legume intake is the most protective dietary predictor of survival among the elderly, regardless of their ethnicity. The study found legumes were associated with long-lived people in various food cultures, such as the Japanese (soy, tofu, and natto), the Swedes (brown beans and peas), and the Mediterranean people (lentils, chickpeas and white beans).[72] Beans and greens are the foods most closely linked in the scientific literature with protection against cancer, diabetes, heart disease, stroke and dementia.

So, stock up on beans and make them your preferred high-carbohydrate food. Most of the soup and stew recipes in *Eat for Health* contain legumes. Add them to a salad to make a filling meal. Dried legumes and beans are a very economical, high-nutrient food.

If you are on a food budget, use lots of dried beans in your cooking and also sprout whole beans and grains for some of your vegetable needs. Soak the whole beans in water overnight in a jar. Strain, rinse and replace the water daily for the next few days, until the sprouts are ready to use.

If beans give you gas or bloating, make sure that you start chewing them very well. It takes some time for your digestive tract to grow the bean-digesting bacteria to digest them better. You may have to start out with a smaller quantity and increase the amount gradually. Don't stop eating beans entirely. It will make things worse when you try to eat them again. Instead, just eat a smaller amount at first, gradually increasing the amount over time.

Nuts, Seeds and Avocado—The Good Fats

High-fat plant foods are high in the essential fatty acids that your body needs. Nuts and seeds and avocado are some of nature's ideal foods for humans and the best source of healthy fats. They can satiate true hunger better than oils because they are rich in critical nutrients and fibers and have one-quarter the calories of an equal amount of oil. They should be part of your healthy eating-style.

Many people perceive raw nuts as high-fat, high-calorie foods that should be avoided or consumed in only token amounts. The important role of raw nuts and seeds in the American diet has been almost completely ignored by nutritional advisers, and their absence is a huge flaw in American cuisine. The results of recent research have changed this perception completely. Today, more and more researchers are finally aware that it is not fat in general that is the villain, but saturated fat, trans fat, and fats consumed in a processed form. The antioxidants and phytochemicals that are in avocados and raw nuts and seeds not only offer unique health benefits, but also maintain the freshness of the food, preventing rancidity of the fat within.

Recent evidence shows that the frequent consumption of nuts is strongly protective against heart disease. An analysis of several large dietary studies found that the people with the highest intake of nuts (about five times per week) had a 39 percent lower risk of coronary heart disease.[73] In addition, several clinical studies have observed beneficial effects of diets high in nuts on lowering cholesterol levels. The beneficial effects of nut consumption observed in clinical and epidemiologic studies underscore the importance of distinguishing between different types of fats. One study estimated that every exchange of one ounce of saturated fat for one ounce of fat from whole nuts was associated with a 45 percent reduction in heart disease risk.[74]

Study after study shows that raw nuts and seeds not only lower cholesterol, but also extend life span and protect against common diseases of aging. They provide a good source of protein, which makes up about 15 to 25 percent of their calories.[75] Their hard shells keep them well protected from pesticides and environmental pollution. Raw nuts and seeds, not the salted or roasted variety, provide the most health benefits.

Over the last few years, the health benefits of seeds also have become more apparent. A tablespoon of ground flax seeds, hemp seeds, chia seeds, or other seeds can supply those hard-to-find omega-3 fats that protect against diabetes, heart disease, and cancer.[76] Seeds are also rich in lignans, a type of fiber associated with a reduced risk of both breast cancer and prostate cancer. In addition, seeds are a good source of iron, zinc, calcium, protein, potassium, magnesium, Vitamin E, and folate. The plant goes to great effort in producing and protecting its seed, filling each genetic package with high concentrations of vitamins, minerals, proteins, essential fats, and enzymes.

While nuts and seeds have great health benefits, they are higher in calories and fat compared to vegetables, beans, and fruits so they should be consumed in smaller amounts. Don't sit in front of the

TV and eat an entire bag of nuts in an hour. Nuts and seeds contain about 175 calories per ounce, and a handful could be a little over one ounce. For most of us, they are not a food that should be eaten in unlimited quantity. Unless you are thin and exercising frequently, hold your consumption of raw nuts and seeds to less than two ounces per day.

Seeds, Nuts and Weight Loss

If you are significantly overweight and want to maximize your weight loss, you should limit your intake of seeds, nuts and avocados to one (one ounce) serving a day since they are calorie-rich. However, you should not exclude these healthy, high-fat foods completely from your diet. Although it may seem illogical to include such high fat foods in your diet (since fat is 9 calories a gram compared with 4 calories a gram for carbohydrates and protein), epidemiological studies show an inverse relationship between seed and nut consumption and body weight. Interestingly, these studies show including some seeds and nuts in your diet actually aids in appetite suppression and weight loss. Well-controlled trials that looked to see if eating nuts and seeds resulted in weight gain found the opposite; eating raw nuts and seeds promoted weight loss, not weight gain.[77]

Because seeds and nuts are rich in minerals and fiber and have a low glycemic index, they are favorable foods to include in a diet designed for diabetics and even the obese. Researchers noted that people eating one ounce of nuts five times a week reduced their risk of developing diabetes by 27 percent.[78]

There is another important reason to include nuts and seeds in your diet as you lose weight. They prevent the formation of gallstones. Weight loss in general can increase one's risk of gallstone formation, but certainly that is a reasonable risk to take when one considers the ill-health and life-threatening effects from significant body fat. It is important to note, as reported in the American Journal of Clinical Nutrition, that when over 80,000 women were followed for 20 years it was found that the regular consumption of nuts and seeds offered dramatic protection against gallstone formation. These findings have also been duplicated in men.[79]

Nuts and seeds should be eaten with meals, not as snacks. When consumed with vegetable-containing meals, they increase absorption of the anticancer phytonutrients. Many of the recipes in this book demonstrate how these disease-fighting foods can be used to make delicious salad dressings and dips.

Eating To Gain Weight

If you are slim or want to gain weight, consuming a larger amount of seeds, nuts and avocado is appropriate. The amount you should consume is based on your body weight, how much fat you have on your body, and how much you exercise. A pregnant or nursing woman should consume about two ounces of seeds and nuts a day, even if overweight, and may consume more than that if slim. A competitive athlete may require four to six ounces or more of raw seeds and nuts a day, in addition to an avocado. In other words, some of us have a higher requirement for these higher-protein, higher-fat foods, and others need less. We do not need as much fat in our diet when we have extra fat on our body that needs to be utilized for energy, but if we are thin (and especially if your physical activity level is high) we may have a substantially higher requirement for fat and calories. Even though we need to consume a significant amount of the lower calorie, very high micronutrient foods, some of these higher calorie foods are also important to fuel our caloric needs.

I provide nutritional counseling to world class and professional athletes to maximize their performance and to increase their resistance to infection. One key feature of the eating-style I recommend to them is that most of their protein and fat needs are met by consuming seeds, nuts, legumes and avocados instead of more animal products. I am not suggesting that these highly active individuals eat a low-fat diet. Rather, it is a diet with lots of healthy, whole-food fats from seeds, nuts and avocados. A diet with fifteen percent of calories from fat could be appropriate for an overweight person with heart disease, but a slim, healthy person may find 30 percent of calories from fat is more appropriate to their needs. A highly active teenager or athlete may function best on a diet that is 40 percent or more of calories from fat. We all should consume a sufficient amount of the highest micronutrient-containing super foods, but consuming seeds, nuts and more starchy vegetables and whole grains may be necessary to meet the requirements of serious athletes with high caloric needs.

Most healthy, normal weight individuals who exercise moderately and are in good shape can eat 3 – 4 ounces of seeds and nuts a day. That will bring their fat intake up to about 30 percent of total calories. Believing fat is the villain is wrong. Eating a bread, potato, and pasta-based diet is not as healthful as a diet higher in fat, where the extra calories (and extra fat and protein) come from seeds and nuts. Eating more beans and whole grains can also be helpful for a person who wants to gain weight. Do not be tempted to eat more animal products to gain weight and don't be deceived by the myth that you need more animal products to build muscle.

Whole Grains
Whole grains include barley, buckwheat (kasha), millet, oats, quinoa, brown rice and wild rice, all of which are high in fiber. Just because a food is called "whole grain" you can't assume it is a good food. Many whole grain cold cereals are so processed that they do not have a significant fiber per serving ratio and have lost most of their nutritional value. The intact (unground) whole grains and the more coarsely ground grains are absorbed into the bloodstream more slowly and they curtail appetite more effectively.

As you know by now, to eat healthfully, fruits and vegetables should form the base of your food pyramid. That means that grains should be consumed in a much smaller amount than you were probably eating before. Grains simply do not contain enough nutrients per calorie to form a substantial part of your diet. You will notice that as you move from Phase 1 to Phase 2 and 3, grain products are gradually reduced.

Many scientific studies show a strong association between the consumption of white flour products, such as pasta and bread and the development of diabetes, obesity, and heart disease.[80] Refined carbohydrates are also linked to enlargement of the prostate.[81] These results continue to show that eating white flour and sweeteners is nutritional suicide.

Whole grains are the least nutrient-dense food of the seed family, and they do not show the powerful protection against disease that is apparent in the scientific studies of fresh fruit, vegetables, beans, raw nuts, or seeds. Just because a food is called whole grain or organic does not make it a good food. Many whole-grain cold cereals are so processed and overly cooked that they have lost most of their nutritional value. Sprouted grains and grains cooked in water are healthier and more nutritious to eat than pre-cooked breakfast cereals. Some of the healthier grains to consume include hulled barley, buckwheat (kasha), millet, oats, quinoa, and wild rice. As a minor part of your diet, they can be water-cooked and used as a breakfast cereal with fruits and nuts or as a dinner side dish.

Animal Products

As you move through this program the goal is to limit animal products to ten percent of caloric intake or less. On the days when you do include animal products in a meal, limit the serving size to under four ounces. Do not make animal products the focus of the meal. Think of them as a garnish or a flavoring agent.

The Level 1 meal plan in this book permits more animal products than I generally recommend. It still is a large reduction in animal product intake for most people and an important first step. If you are comfortable eating fewer animal products in Level One, go for it. Full-fat dairy, such as cheese and butter, are the foods with the highest saturated fat content, so choose fat-free dairy products, and for the same reason, try to choose white meat fowl, fish and eggs. Avoid processed meats, luncheon meats, bacon, hot dogs, and any pickled, darkened, blackened, barbecued or overcooked animal products.

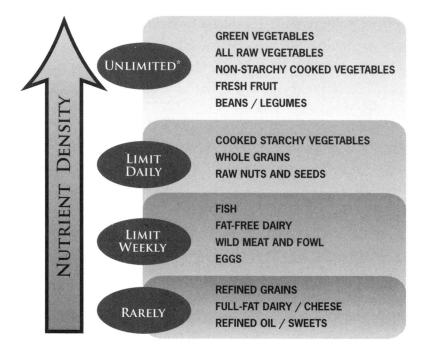

* Unlimited based on not overeating

Keep in mind that eating to maintain extra fat stores on your body, because you or others think you look better heavier, is never healthful. A healthy person is slim and muscular. If you think you are too thin and desire more weight on your frame, the right way to achieve that is from working out in the gym, not in the kitchen. The muscular demands on your body will then increase your appetite, hunger will occur more frequently, and your caloric intake will increase proportionally to the increased muscular demand. If you want to gain weight, try to make your thighs, shoulders and chest a little bigger with more exercise. Don't expand your waistline by over-exercising your knife and fork.

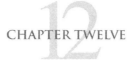

CHAPTER TWELVE

EXERCISES WITH FOOD: THE ADVANCED WORKOUT

It's time for some advanced exercises with food. As you already know from the previous ones that you have been doing, these food activities can help increase the pleasure you derive from natural food, which will help you adjust to eating with the goal of superior nutrition. Like all exercises, they require frequent practice in order to see results. Continue doing the previous exercises with a particular focus on stretching the palate. This will help you rid yourself of toxic hunger.

HERE ARE THREE ADVANCED EXERCISES FOR YOU.

EXERCISE 5

Make a point to eat a light lunch or a light breakfast each day. Eating one lighter meal without snacking before the next meal, either lunch or dinner, will increase your true hunger before that meal. Over time, this will help to teach you what true hunger feels like. The main exercise target here is to see if you can get back in touch with the sensations of "true hunger," differentiating them from the sensations of "toxic hunger." Be patient because it may take some time for toxic hunger to go away. It will help if you can link together an entire week of superior nutrition so that you lose the toxic hunger symptoms and begin the pleasurable sensation of true hunger.

EXERCISE 6

Reduce your consumption of animal products (meat, eggs, dairy products) to no more than one serving per day, then push yourself further and do not use animal products more than one serving every other day. Use the high vegetable recipes in this book to replace animal products in your menus.

EXERCISE 7

Remove white flour, sugar and other sweeteners from your diet. This means using fewer refined, processed foods. Store-purchased products should be 100 percent whole grain and contain no sweetening agents.

Adopting a high-nutrient diet is a big change for most people, but clearly it is not an all-or-nothing plan. It is a journey toward taking control of your health destiny. No matter what phase or level you start with, positive changes will provide rewards. Have fun, enjoy your food and *eat for health*.

WORK OUT PERFORMANCE GOALS

1. Continue doing the Exercises from previous chapters.

2. Eat a light breakfast or lunch and learn to experience the feeling of "true" hunger.

3. Greatly reduce animal products (meat, fish, dairy) in your diet.

4. Eliminate or greatly reduce refined, processed foods made with white sugar and white flour.

How will I be different two years from now?

_____

_____

_____

_____

_____

_____

_____

_____

TODAYS DATE _____

Two Years from now:

_____

_____

_____

_____

_____

_____

_____

_____

_____

_____

CHAPTER THIRTEEN

THREE COMPONENTS OF HEALTH

"After three heart attacks within three months of each other and five angioplasties in a three-year period, I was still very ill. I almost died soon after the last angioplasty and had internal bleeding that was difficult to stop. The torture of all my medical problems made me think I would be better off if I had died. I was left with unstable angina, meaning I had chest pain from my bad heart almost constantly. I weighed 225 pounds and I could not walk one block. I was on ten medications and I was a cardiac cripple at the age of 60.

Luckily, I learned about Dr. Fuhrman and read his book, *Eat To Live*. Within three months of following the plan, my chest pain was gone, and I was walking again. From not being able to walk one block, I was able to walk two miles with no problems. Within seven months of eating Dr. Fuhrman's high-nutrient density plan, I weighed 135 pounds. I just wanted to be healthier and live again, but, in doing so, I had lost 90 pounds without even trying to lose weight.

When I think back to how sick I was, it is frightening. In addition to my other ailments, I suffered from daily migraines and had bleeding ulcers from all the medications I took. Now I walk three miles a day, go to yoga, exercise, and enjoy life immensely. I know I would not be alive today if not for Dr. Fuhrman's plan."

Julia Spano
Colonia, New Jersey

If you felt compelled to begin this journey, it was likely instinct that was driving you. Every living organism has a built-in instinct to survive and to thrive. As you continue on the path towards maximizing your health, you will reach the point where this type of nutrient-rich eating will become second nature. By being consistent in putting your newly obtained knowledge into practice, it will become ingrained as your healthful, new way of living. If you have been doing the food exercises I have recommended, you are probably already feeling a lot better than before and have the desire to feel even better.

In these final chapters, I will be giving you additional information to help you continue on your path to great health. Many people invest in their financial future but never consider their health future. The way you take care of yourself is just as crucial a determinant of your future happiness as your savings account. A large nest egg is of no use to you if you're not here to spend it!

As you plan for your health future, you must consider the three important components that pay you back with high returns: your nutritional, physical, and social states. Each factor must be considered:

- NUTRITIONAL COMPONENT — Make every calorie count as you strive for maximum nutrition. Remember my health equation, H = N/C. Strive to eat foods that have high ANDI scores. Become a Nutritarian!

- PHYSICAL COMPONENT — Make physical exercise a part of your normal routine. Joining a gym is a great bonus, but learn to exploit all of the other opportunities in your life to exercise your body during the normal course of the day. Take the stairs instead of the elevator. When possible, walk instead of ride. Once you embrace nutritional excellence, you can strive for physical excellence. You may find that exercise becomes easier and more pleasurable with better health and lower weight.

- SOCIAL COMPONENT — Build a strong mental defense against unhealthy influences. A healthy mindset is a prerequisite for a healthy lifestyle, and the best way to develop one is to be optimistic and surround yourself with people who engage in and support your health. Even if you don't feel naturally optimistic, you can learn the attitude. Just reading this book shows you are optimistic.

These three factors are all healthful habits that will eventually become second nature. The more you do them, the more they become your preferred way of life. Many unhealthy and healthy people are obsessed with food. Eating the right foods will make you incredibly healthy, but avoid obsessions even with healthy foods. They are often indicators of compulsions and other social issues. Striking a balance between eating and not eating is an excellent way to eliminate the obsession and strive for a fully balanced life where people, food, pleasure, recreation, exercise, work, rest, and sleep all have their place. The key to finding food's place in this balance is making the material you're learning instinctive and a natural part of your life.

Addictions also make attempts at dietary modifications more difficult, but it only takes a few seconds of decision-making to win the battle and say an emphatic "no" to the addiction and "yes" to your new healthful lifestyle. I want to mention again that I have observed thousands of cases in which these positive changes have resulted in some temporary discomfort as the body eliminates toxins and restores its cells to a more youthful, decongested state. This is normal, and coping with it on the road to better health will be a small price to pay. By now, some change has certainly occurred in your life as a result of learning this body of knowledge and beginning to eat a nutrient-dense diet.

Do not underestimate the human body's powerful capacity for self-healing when superior nutrition has been established and dietary and emotional stresses are removed. Many people have made these changes and have completely recovered from chronic illnesses that their doctors told them they would have forever.

During most of human history, getting adequate calories was a difficult struggle. In those days, malnutrition from food scarcity was the major problem, not obesity. Humans are able to survive in so many environments because we are the most adaptable species on the planet. Now, our adaptability has become a liability because unhealthful options have become so accessible. However, you can control the choices that you make. This book is about change and restoration. Hopefully, it will spur you to confront your fears about different dietary choices, reclaim your natural tastes, and restore your natural hunger drive.

The Stubborn Habits

You've learned which foods are best for your body, and you've been practicing high-nutrient eating so you know that you can eat most healthful foods to your heart's content. It sounds like all your food problems are solved. Or are they? Do you still crave foods that you know are bad for you even when you aren't hungry? Let's talk briefly again about addiction and how to get beyond it.

Modern foods are designed to seduce your taste buds. You have been manipulated by profit-motivated food manufacturers. We all have. The artificially concentrated flavors that the processed food industry uses to stimulate the brain's pleasure center are designed to increase and retain sales. Processed and refined foods entice us to eat even when we are not truly hungry. Tragically, the result is that they lead people's taste buds astray. Artificial, intense flavors cause us to enjoy natural flavors less. Our taste buds become desensitized, and the more we succumb to the heightened, artificial flavors, the less appealing natural, whole foods become. As we have discussed, salt also desensitizes our taste buds, we need more and more to experience any pleasurable sensation.

Fortunately, by practicing this high-nutrient diet, your sensory abilities will start bouncing back. It might take more time to reset your receptors to appreciate the more subtle flavors of whole, unprocessed foods. Hang in there, and keep up your healthful eating! It's the only way for this to happen, and it always does. It might take longer than six weeks, but your taste and flavor sensitivity will improve tremendously over time.

Realizing your impediments and gaining knowledge about great health are tremendous first steps, but they are only half of the overall solution. You must put into practice and repeat your new beneficial behaviors over and over until they become part of you. Repetition will make these positive actions feel more and more natural. The more you make healthful meals, and the more days you link together eating healthful foods, the more your brain will naturally prefer to eat this way.

Developing a burning desire for optimal health will help you in this process. Stay with the program and you will cease to crave flavor enhancers and highly seasoned food. You will gradually transform into a person who actually prefers to eat this way. You will stop craving the junk foods that have been destroying your health. Trying the recipes contained in this book will help you learn how to make better food choices. For example, my healthy sorbets and ice creams are the perfect substitutes for the frozen desserts you may currently crave.

It is not easy to develop new habits, and there is no such thing as a quick shortcut to developing new skills and expertise. However, if you are motivated to persevere and keep trying, it becomes easier. Feeling better and losing weight are great motivators. Don't give up. The only failure is to stop trying.

Planning and Exercise

The ability to consistently make good decisions requires good planning. You need time to prepare your environment so that you have good-tasting, healthy foods around you at all times to minimize temptation. Because eating healthfully has only gained popularity in recent years, few restaurants or fast-food places make eating this way convenient. And because most of us work, it can be tough to fit everything, including cooking and exercise, into our busy schedules. Therefore, if you are going to succeed at turning your health or weight around, you will need to organize your time.

This book is not about exercise, but it is still important to mention that, without regular exercise, you cannot expect great health benefits. For excellent health in our later years, excellent nutrition must go hand in hand with regular, rigorous exercise. Our muscles and bones will shrink and weaken as we age if we do not exercise regularly and place demands on our skeleton. Osteoporosis is mostly the result of a sedentary lifestyle.

If you shop and cook twice each week, you can still have time to exercise on the other days. Plenty of people exercise four times per week by following a schedule such as this: exercise once on Saturday, once on Sunday, and then two more times during the week. Below is a sample of a schedule of eating plans and exercising that you can modify for your own needs.

SAMPLE WEEKLY SCHEDULE		
Saturday	Eat out or take out food or salad bar	Exercise A
Sunday	Shop and cook today	Exercise B
Monday	Eat leftovers	day off
Tuesday	Eat leftovers	Exercise A
Wednesday	Shop and cook today	day off
Thursday	Eat leftovers	Exercise B
Friday	Eat leftovers	day off

EXERCISE A DAYS:

Walk uphill on an incline treadmill, skip rope, or ride a bike; plus work out your abs, lower back and chest. Even fifteen minutes of heart-beat-elevating, calorie-burning cardio, such as walking on a steep incline or pedaling on an elliptical machine, is good. If using a treadmill, gradually increase the incline as your cardiovascular fitness and exercise tolerance improves.

EXERCISE B DAYS

Exercise on an elliptical machine or a stair-climber; plus work out legs, biceps, triceps, latissmus dorsi, and trapezius with weights or resistance. Aim for some cardio activities with an elevated pulse four times a week.

Make a list of all the exercises that you like to do and separate them into two different workouts. For example, make the A exercise day easier on the thighs and B exercise day heavier on the thighs so that you will be able to handle the B exercise day, even if it is the next day, without having your legs feel too tired.

Your exercise schedule and what exercises or activities you do should be individualized to your needs and preferences. The underlying theme is to plan it into your schedule. Do not exercise the same body parts on consecutive days, and spread out many different exercises to encompass various body parts into your weekly plan. If you are new to exercise, start slowly so you do not injure yourself. Begin by walking on a tread mill with only a three or four degree incline and lifting some very light dumbbells. Over time, keep increasing the incline on the treadmill, so you can eventually perform a more vigorous workout and burn more calories in your time allotment. Only increase speed on the treadmill after your increasing fitness level has enabled you to perform comfortably at the highest incline. It is better to go slower at a higher incline, than go faster at a lower incline. It puts less stress on your joints and you burn more calories.

If you belong to a fitness facility or have access to a fitness professional, inquire about other exercises and the proper form of your workouts. Don't push yourself too hard, but make sure that you are doing physical exercise at least three times per week.

If you are significantly overweight, diabetic or have heart disease and your capacity for vigorous exercise is low, you will need to exercise more frequently, even two or three times a day. The lower your fitness level and the lower the intensity of exercise that you are capable of, the more frequently you need to exercise. Many of my patients with diabetes exercise twice daily. It is like their medicine before lunch and dinner. Even ten minutes of exercise, done regularly, is better than no exercise.

The more thoroughly you plan your weekly schedule in advance, the easier it will be to ingrain your new habits into your life. We live busy lives, we work hard, and we have to plan even our recreational activities and vacations in advance.

So, make a weekly health plan and figure out:

- When are you going to shop?

- What you are going to purchase when you shop? Be sure to make a list!

- What dishes, soups, or dressings are you going to prepare when you cook?

- What dishes are you going to make in large volume to store in the refrigerator or freezer and use on multiple days?

- What frozen veggies and fruits are you are going to have on hand?

- When are you going to exercise?

- What exercises or activities are you going to do?

- When will you go to sleep and wake up?

- How many relaxation, entertainment, and social activities can you plan to fit in?

Remember, not only does regular exercise burn calories during the time you are actually exercising, it also increases the caloric needs of your body into the days ahead, even on the days you are not exercising. It will work with your new eating-style to deliver dramatic benefits. Exercise is the only way to increase your metabolic rate, healthfully.

CHAPTER FOURTEEN

SNACKING, SHOPPING AND EATING OUT

Eliminate Temptation

Most people agree that they make better food choices if they make a point of eliminating temptations. It is best if you can get rid of all the unhealthy food in your kitchen. If it isn't in the house, you won't be faced with the constant question of whether or not to eat it. This strategy can be one of the most important steps toward healthful living. Eventually, healthy food will taste just as good as unhealthful options. You just have to learn the best ways to prepare it and how to get your taste buds in shape to enjoy it.

If your family does not want to join your health makeover, then create a separate area in the pantry and refrigerator for your foods. It is more challenging if you have to make unhealthy foods for your family while you're in the midst of your own health makeover, but don't let the obstacles stop you. Remember, by making yourself healthier and enjoying it, you are opening the door for others to potentially follow your lead. Share what you are learning and your excitement about your changes, and let each person come to their own conclusions in their own time. It is very likely that when your family and friends see you looking and feeling better, they will want to know more about what you are doing, and you will eventually have others join you on your quest for better health.

Try Not to Snack

For maximum success, it is best to eat only when you are hungry and to stop eating as soon as you feel satisfied. This will require less willpower as you progress and get better at meeting your body's nutritional and volume requirements. I want you to try to get back in touch with your body's signals. Try to eat only when you feel hungry and as time progresses, pay attention to see if you can develop the ability to distinguish true hunger—felt in the throat—from the symptoms of toxic hunger. Remember, the symptoms of toxic hunger, which are caused by withdrawal, won't turn off until you have provided your body with adequate nutrients and your body has had time to build up a nutrient reserve in its tissues. This could take a few weeks to a few months, so be patient.

Eating when hungry usually translates into a three meal-per-day format, without snacking. Unless you are a dedicated athlete or a physical laborer, you probably don't burn enough calories to justify snacking. Snacking is most often recreational eating, without true hunger present. It has negative effects, including the following:

1) usually results in the consumption of higher amounts of calories each week.

2) prevents you from experiencing true hunger before meals, thus diminishing enjoyment of food.

3) prevents your digestive tract from getting the rest it needs to build up digestive enzymes for proper digestion.

4) less efficient detoxification and cellular repair.

Animal studies have shown that eating less frequently results in increased life span. The healthier you eat, the quicker the desire to eat between meals and the symptoms of toxic hunger will disappear.

Some helpful hints to combat snacking are:

- Eat a salad or raw vegetables with a dip to start both lunch and dinner.

- Keep lots of frozen fruits and vegetables and pre-washed fresh foods in your home.

- Have cooked greens or soups with greens at every lunch and dinner.

- Don't eat after 8:00 p.m.

- Have a fruit sorbet or fruit dessert after dinner and then clean the kitchen, clean your teeth, and end eating for the day.

Food Shopping

Your health makeover will require some brushing up on your shopping skills. It's easy to shop for high-nutrient foods; they are mostly in the produce aisle. Since it is necessary to consume a variety of fresh fruits and vegetables, I recommend that you shop twice a week. You will use the main shopping trip of the week to stock up on staples and produce for three or four days. Your second trip of the week can be a short trip to restock fresh fruits and vegetables. You will spend most of your time in the produce, health food, and frozen food sections. The supermarket is filled with temptation, so try to avoid certain aisles. The center aisles of most stores contain the most heavily processed foods, so consider them non-existent and do not travel down those aisles. What you don't see can't tempt you!

You can use all spices and herbs except for salt. When using condiments, mustard is okay if unsalted mustard is an available option, but pickled foods contain too much salt and should be avoided. If you love ketchup or tomato sauce, look for low sodium or no-salt-added options.

Reading Food Labels

I want you to read food labels, but you'll get the best dietary outcomes if you try to avoid foods that have labels. With the exception of unprocessed frozen fruits and vegetables, foods that come in boxes, bags and jars are usually highly processed and low in nutrients-per-calorie. When you buy foods that have labels, be selective and use good judgment. If you know what to look for and how to interpret it, food labels can help you evaluate the healthfulness of a product. Don't be misled by the other writing on the package. It is essentially advertising, and tells you little, if anything, about the nutritional content of the product. The ingredient list contains the most important information. It is often in very small print and difficult to find and read, but read it you must. Inspect the label before you add an item to your shopping cart.

Reading labels reinforces the idea that you need to put most products back on the shelf. Avoid foods that list white flour (often called wheat flour) and any type of sweetener, such as corn syrup, among the first few ingredients. Ingredients are listed on the label according to quantity, in descending order based on weight (from most to least). As a general rule of thumb, if the list of ingredients is long and you cannot pronounce most of them, there are probably a lot of chemical additives in the product, and you're risking your health by eating it.

Be sure to read the ingredients even when purchasing foods from a health food store or when the rest of the packaging is trying to convince you the food is healthy. For example, watch out for statements like these on packages:

- NATURAL FRUIT FLAVORS

- WITH REAL FRUIT JUICE

- ALL NATURAL INGREDIENTS

- NO ARTIFICIAL PRESERVATIVES

- 100% NATURAL

- REAL FRUIT

- NO PRESERVATIVES

- NO ARTIFICIAL INGREDIENTS

Statements like these do not mean there are no harmful additives in the product or that the products are healthful. They simply mean the manufacturer hopes you'll think there are no harmful ingredients. For example, here is the list of ingredients from a loaf of bread that claims, 'ALL NATURAL INGREDIENTS,' and 'NO ARTIFICIAL PRESERVATIVES ADDED,' on its label:

Enriched wheat flour (wheat flour, malted barley, niacin, reduced iron, thiamine mononitrate, riboflavin), water, high fructose corn syrup, yeast, wheat bran, vital wheat gluten, butter. Contains 2% or less of each of the following: rye meal, corn flour, molasses, rolled whole wheat, salt, dough conditioners (ammonium sulfate, sodium stearoyl lactylate), brown sugar, honey, vinegar, oatmeal, soy flour, mono and diglycerides, partially hydrogenated soybean oil.

As you read this list, notice that the first two ingredients listed are white flour and sugar. This bread is junk food.

- Enriched wheat flour is white flour. The bran and the germ portion of the whole wheat, which are rich in vitamins and minerals, have been removed. To compensate for refining out approximately twenty nutrients, four are added back. Use only products made with whole wheat flour, it must have the word "whole" on the label.

- High fructose corn syrup is a concentrated form of sugar derived from corn.

- Dough conditioners, in general, can cause mineral deficiencies, and ammonium sulfate in particular may cause mouth ulcers, nausea, and kidney and liver problems.

- Brown sugar is merely white sugar with molasses added.

- Partially hydrogenated soybean oil is a trans fat associated with heart disease, breast and colon cancer, atherosclerosis and elevated cholesterol. It is even worse than saturated fat.

As you can see, this "all-natural" bread will not help you on your road to health. Even if you didn't know the particular detriments of each ingredient, taking the time to read that it's main ingredients are white flour and sugar, and that the rest of the list is lengthy, would tell you to leave it on the shelf.

When looking at labels, we also need to be aware of sodium levels. A lot of sodium is "hidden" in processed foods from spaghetti sauce to canned soup to frozen dinners. Obviously, if you see the word "salt" on a food label, you know salt is in the product. But baking soda and monosodium glutamate (MSG) contain sodium, too. To avoid excess sodium, try to avoid products with: brine, disodium phosphate, garlic salt, onion salt, sodium alginate, sodium benzoate, sodium caseinate, sodium citrate, sodium hydroxide, sodium nitrate, sodium pectinate, sodium proprionate, and sodium sulfite. Also avoid anything using the words "pickled," "cured," "broth," and "soy sauce." They all indicate high sodium.

Just because a product says that it has reduced sodium or is light in sodium, it does not mean it is a low sodium product. It only means it has less than the higher sodium version of the product. Lots of these products still contain much too much salt for good health.

IF THE LABEL SAYS...	IT MEANS...
Sodium free/salt free	Less than 5 mg sodium added per serving
Very low sodium	Less than 35 mg sodium added per serving
Low sodium	Less than 140 mg sodium per serving
Reduced sodium	At least 25% less sodium than the original product
Light in sodium	At least 50% less sodium than the original product
Unsalted / No added salt	No salt added during processing (not necessarily sodium-free)

You want to keep your overall daily sodium intake under 1200 mg and preferably under 1000 mg. Natural foods contain less than 0.5 mg of sodium per calorie. If a serving of food provides 100 calories and it contains 400 mg of sodium, then you know it had plenty of salt added to it. Since you get 400-700 mg of sodium daily from natural whole foods, you don't want processed foods to push you over the limit. Be sure to read the food labels, and do not add more than 200-400 mg of extra sodium per day, so you don't push yourself up over that 1000-1200 mg limit.

In addition to sodium, most processed foods contain a litany of food additives with toxic properties. Substances such as artificial colors, sweeteners, stabilizers, nitrates, and preservatives often are linked to cancer in lab animals and may be harmful or cancer promoting in humans. They are best avoided.

Lets take a look at a sample food label to discover what else we can learn from this packaging.

SAMPLE LABEL FOR MACARONI & CHEESE

① Start Here →

② Check Calories →

③ Limit these Nutrients →

④ Get Enough of these Nutrients →

⑤ Footnote →

Nutrition Facts

Serving Size 1 cup (228g)
Servings Per Container 2

Amount Per Serving

Calories 250   Calories from Fat 110

	% Daily Value*
Total Fat 12g	**18%**
Saturated Fat 3g	**15%**
Trans Fat 3g	
Cholesterol 30g	**10%**
Sodium 470mg	**20%**
Total Carbohydrate 31g	**10%**
Dietary Fiber 0g	**0%**
Sugars 5g	
Protein 5g	
Vitamin A	**4%**
Vitamin C	**2%**
Calcium	**20%**
Iron	**4%**

* Percent Daily Values are based on a 2,000 calorie diet.
Your Daily Values may be higher or lower depending on
your calorie needs.

	Calories:	2,000	2,500
Total Fat	Less than	65g	80g
Sat Fat	Less than	20g	25g
Cholesterol	Less than	300mg	300mg
Sodium	Less than	2,400mg	2,400mg
Total Carbohydrate		300g	375g
Dietary Fiber		25g	30g

The Serving Size

Serving Size 1 cup (228g)
Servings Per Container 2

The first place to start when you look at the Nutrition Facts label is the serving size and the number of servings in the package. Serving sizes are standardized to make it easier to compare similar foods; they are provided in familiar units, such as cups or pieces, followed by the metric amount, e.g., the number of grams. The size of the serving on the food package influences the number of calories and the nutrient amounts listed on the top part of the label. Pay attention to the serving size, especially how many servings there are in the food package. The serving size might not be what you or any other consumer typically eats in a serving.

 Calories
(and Calories from Fat)

Amount Per Serving

Calories 250   Calories from Fat 110

Remember, the main focus of the *Eat For Health* program is not the number of calories, but the quality of calories. It is the amount of nutrients per calorie that determines the quality of the calories. Eating low-nutrient calories is not only linked to being overweight and becoming diabetic, but it is also a chief cause of heart disease and cancer.

Total Fat 12g	18%
Saturated Fat 3g	15%
Trans Fat 3g	
Cholesterol 30g	10%
Sodium 470mg	20%

The nutrients listed first are the ones Americans generally eat in excess amounts. Eating processed food can give us extra saturated fat, cholesterol, and sodium, but a serious problem in processed food can also be the trans fat or hydrogenated oils. Ignore the percentage recommendations because they are overly permissive. Eating according to those can take 20 or 30 years off your life from a heart attack or a stroke. Avoid processed foods that are high in sodium, meaning they contain over 300 mg of sodium per serving.

4

Dietary Fiber 0g	0%
Sugars 5g	
Protein 5g	
Vitamin A	4%
Vitamin C	2%
Calcium	20%
Iron	4%

Most Americans don't get enough dietary fiber, vitamins, and minerals from their diet. You might want to look for foods that contain more of the nutrients on the label, but because the list of nutrients is so narrow, it's not really helpful. When you focus on only a few nutrients, it can make a food look satisfactory when it actually contains a very narrow complement of nutrients. The little bit of nutrients in or added to processed foods can be confusing. For example, Cocoa Puffs and Fruit Loops have some nutrients added to them to make their labels look better, but these are not healthy foods. The range of nutrients added back to these and other processed foods is too narrow and the level of phytochemicals is too low. Natural foods not only contain larger amounts of these basic nutrients, but also contain thousands of phytochemicals that have never even been named. Since this short list of nutrients that manufacturers provide is not helpful, it makes sense to ignore it.

QUICK GUIDE TO READING LABELS:

- Food labels list ingredients in descending order. What's first on the ingredient list is present in the highest quantity.

- Do not purchase foods that contain white flour (also written as wheat flour) or sweeteners in the first four ingredients or that contain any hydrogenated (trans) fat, or chemical additives.

- Avoid foods with more mg of sodium than the amount of calories in the serving size.

Eating in Restaurants

Dining out can be challenging when transitioning to a high-nutrient diet. The first step when going out to eat is trying to find a restaurant that will have some healthful options. Many restaurants will cater to your needs and preferences. Call ahead and ask. Eat early before the restaurant gets very crowded so the staff will have time to modify a dish or make something for you.

If your restaurant meal is a breakfast, stay away from the bread, bagels, and breakfast sweets. It is easy to find oatmeal, fruit or eggs.

For lunch and dinner, ask for an extra side of steamed vegetables instead of pasta or white rice to accompany your main dish. Patronize restaurants that have salad bars. You can also order Asian vegetable dishes that are steamed or water sautéed with the dressing or sauce on the side. Because soups are made in advance in restaurants and are always very high in salt, it is best that you do not eat soups when you are out. Stick with salads and a main dish. I often order a double-sized salad and let them charge me double. I often order a double-sized portion of whatever green vegetable they have fresh, adding, "Can you make that without oil, salt or butter:" Then I add the vegetables to my salad.

Ask the waiter not to bring bread to the table, so you are not tempted to fill up before the meal. Always order the salad dressing on the side so you can use their high-salt dressings sparingly. You can also ask if they have olive oil to use instead of butter on potatoes or to use (with or without vinegar) instead of the high-salt salad dressing.

The more you practice, the better you will get at handling all of the many eating situations that arise. Remember, the goal is not to eat perfectly at every single meal. The goal is to eat very well the vast majority of the time. If you eat an unhealthful meal, don't despair; just start eating healthfully again at your next meal.

HELPFUL HINT:

Eating too quickly encourages overeating and can tax the digestive system. It takes about 15 minutes for your brain to realize that your stomach is full. If you eat too fast, your body won't have enough time to tell you when it's full. You will end up eating more than you really needed. Slow down, thoroughly chew your food, and enjoy the experience of eating. Don't just grab food without thinking about it.

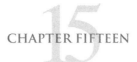
COOKING TECHNIQUES AND TIPS

As you continue to learn more about my healthy cooking techniques and delicious recipes, here are some guidelines you should concentrate on to assure you are eating a high-nutrient diet:

BASIC NUTRITARIAN GUIDELINES

1. Eat a large raw salad each day. The amount of leafy lettuce and other leafy greens such as spinach and arugula in the salad should amount to at least five ounces. If you want to jump up to a higher level of excellence, double this quantity of leafy greens.

2. Add other raw vegetables (besides the leafy greens) such as tomatoes, shredded carrots, cabbage, beets, snow peas, or raw broccoli to the salad so the total amount of raw vegetables for the day amounts to at least 12 ounces of food.

3. Consume a double-portion serving of steamed green vegetables (at least twelve ounces a day). Vegetables such as asparagus, artichokes, kale, collards, broccoli, Brussels sprouts, string beans, baby bok choy, and others should be eaten every day. You can also do this by adding these greens to a soup.

4. Eat between one-half cup and one cup of beans daily in a vegetable soup, on your salad, as an ingredient to a main dish or in a dip.

5. Eat at least one ounce of raw seeds or nuts daily, preferably in one of the delicious salad dressings or dips which are featured in the recipe section. Try to use more seeds and less nuts.

6. Eat at least three fresh fruits daily. Try to eat some berries, cherries or other high-nutrient fruits regularly.

7. Have some fresh squeezed vegetable juice either by itself or part of your soup base on most days.

8. Measure and control the type and amount of animal products consumed. Do not eat more than four servings of animal products per week and limit the size of the portion so it is under four ounces (about the size of a deck of cards). As you gain experience, try to reduce the amount of animal products you eat even further. It would be a significant health achievement if you do not have more than two or three servings of animal products each week. In other words, whether you have two eggs, chicken in your salad or soup, or a turkey sandwich on whole grain pita, make the next day a strict vegetarian day. Keep full-fat dairy very limited and do not eat processed, barbecued or salted meats.

9. Reduce and measure your salt intake. Do not cook with salt in the home. Do not eat soup or sauces in restaurants; they are too high in sodium. Always order the dressing on the side and ask if the food can be prepared without the sauce. If you are using a packaged or third-party prepared food, make sure

the sodium content per serving is the same or lower than the calories. When just starting out, make 400 mg per serving the most you ever eat, and make sure that this is the only sodium-extra food that you consume that day.

10. Get most of your starch intake from carrots, peas, sweet potato, squash and beans, not from flour products and white potato. Do not eat white flour products. If you're using bread and pasta, use limited amounts, not more than one serving per day and, of course, make sure it is 100 percent whole grain.

11. Limit your consumption of oil to no more than one tablespoon daily. Oil is a fattening, low-nutrient food. If you eat something cooked with oil, make sure you do not use oil on your salad that day.

12. Use the ANDI scores in Chapter Three to help you make the most nutrient-dense food choices.

Knowing how and what to eat is one thing; actually doing it is another. Making great tasting, high-nutrient meals is the best way to overcome any temptation to fall back on old unhealthful eating habits.

HELPFUL TOOLS

Your journey to excellent health will be much easier if you have all of the tools you need in your kitchen. You may already have everything you need to start cooking, but take a few minutes to make sure you are supplied with these important basics:

- Food chopper or a good knife set

- Wok with cover or large pan with cover

- Pressure cooker — Steaming vegetables with a pressure cooker preserves more nutrients than regular steaming because the vegetables can be softened in a significantly shorter cooking time, with less water and without excessive heat.

- High-powered blender — Some of the recipes in this book require a powerful blender. Even though it's an expensive piece of equipment, it is well worth the investment because it produces smooth and creamy salad dressings, dips, smoothies, sorbets and blended salads. It is ideal for pureeing vegetables and nuts into soup and grinding nuts and seeds. The Vitamix brand blender is a good choice.

- Vegetable juicer — Fresh squeezed juice is more flavorful than canned or bottled juice. Using freshly juiced carrots in my soup recipes that call for carrot juice will optimize the flavor of these recipes.

  A juicer is different from a blender. When fruits or vegetables are put into a blender, the end product contains everything that went into the blender, but a juicer will separate the juice from the pulp. With juicing, you retain many of the phytochemicals and other nutrients, but lose some beneficial components like fiber.

HELPFUL HINT:

Some people have difficulty digesting large quantities of roughage when they first switch to a natural plant-based diet. Often problems with gas and bloating can be solved by replacing some whole raw and cooked fruits and vegetables with blended dishes. Juicing is also a good way to supplement nutrient intake while the body is adjusting to higher fiber levels.

COOKING TECHNIQUES

There are a few essential cooking techniques that are used in many of the recipes in this book.

Water Sautéing

Water sautéing (also called sweating or steam frying) is used instead of cooking with oil. Water sautéing is simple and easy to use for stir-fries, sauces, and many other dishes. To water sauté, heat a skillet, wok or pan on high heat until water sputters when dropped on the pan. Add a small amount of water and when hot, add the vegetables and cook, covering occasionally and adding more water as necessary until tender. Do not add too much water, or the food will be boiled not sautéed. To develop flavor in the onions, garlic or other vegetables you are cooking, let the pan get dry enough for the food to start to brown just a little before you add additional water.

Soups and Stews

When we steam or boil vegetables, many of the beneficial phytochemicals, vitamins and minerals are transferred to the water and lost. Soups and stews play a big role in my diet-style because when vegetables are simmered in a soup, all the nutrients are retained in the liquid.

Soups and stews are cooked at 212° F, the boiling point of water. Cooking at this low temperature is very healthful because no acrylamides are produced. Acrylamides are the cancer-causing agents formed during high temperature cooking such as frying, baking, roasting and grilling.

Many of the soup recipes use fresh vegetable juices, especially carrot juice to provide a great tasting, antioxidant-rich base. Juice your own carrots for maximum flavor or if you are short of time, bottled carrot and other vegetable juices can be purchased. Low-sodium V8 is another option to add to the soup base. No-salt-added or low sodium vegetable broth is also used in some soup recipes.

To make a "cream" soup, raw cashews or cashew butter can be blended into the soup to provide a creamy texture and rich flavor. In many of my recipes, a portion of the cooked soup is removed from the pot, and blended with raw cashews. This blended portion is then added back to the pot.

A big advantage to making soups and stews is that they are great leftovers. Soups generally keep well for up to four days in the refrigerator, but should be frozen if longer storage is desirable. Be creative with your soup making. Once you get the general idea, you can mix and match ingredients. Start with a base like carrot juice, low-sodium tomato juice or vegetable broth. Add some leafy greens, a member of the onion family, some flavoring like Vegi-Zest and any other vegetables that you have on hand. Don't forget the beans! Create new soups by matching up different items from the columns in the following chart.

HELPFUL HINT:

If you choose to occasionally use a prepared soup keep in mind that you want your overall daily sodium intake to remain under 1000 -1200 mg. You get around 400 to 800 mg of sodium from natural whole foods, so you want to keep the sodium you consume from processed foods below 200-400 mg per day. You will be amazed how much sodium canned soup contains. Be sure to read the labels.

SOUPS AND STEWS – THE NUTRITARIAN WAY

Base	Leafy Greens	Allum Family	Other Veggies	Flavor	Beans
Carrot Juice	Kale	Onion	Fresh or Dried Tomato	Dr. Fuhrman's VegiZest or MatoZest	Cannellini or other White Beans
Low Sodium or No Salt Added Vegetable Broth	Spinach	Leek	Mushrooms	Basil, Cilantro, Parsley or Dill	Red Kidney
Low Sodium Tomato Juice	Collards or Mustard Greens	Garlic	Red or Green Bell Pepper	Thyme, Oregano, Rosemary, Sage, Marjoram	Lentils or Split Peas
Celery Juice	Swiss Chard	Shallots	Broccoli	Bay Leaves	Black Beans
Low Sodium V-8	Bok Choy	Ginger	Sweet Potato	Chili Powder, Cumin	Garbanzo Beans (Chick Peas)
Beet Juice	Cabbage		Carrots and Celery	Curry Powder	Navy Beans
			Zucchini, Butternut Squash, Acorn Squash	Lemon or Lime	Edamame or Tofu
			Parsnips	Cayenne or Hot Pepper Flakes	

HOW TO COOK BEANS

Most dried beans should be soaked overnight before cooking. If you forgot to soak them overnight, use the quick-soak method: In a large saucepan, cover dried beans with triple their volume of cold water (for example 3 cups of water for 1 cup of beans). Bring water to a boil and cook beans uncovered, over moderate heat 2 minutes. Remove pan from heat and soak beans 1 hour.

After soaking, bring beans to a boil, and then lower the heat to a simmer. Most beans require about one and a half to two hours of cooking. Lentils and split peas require one hour and do not need to be soaked prior to cooking. Make sure beans are thoroughly cooked, as they are more difficult to digest when undercooked.

Beans may also be cooked in a pressure cooker to reduce cooking time. Put the beans in the pressure cooker with 3 times as much water as beans. Cook at 15 pounds pressure for 30 minutes for small beans and about 40 minutes for large beans.

Use this guide to determine how much dried beans to cook:

1/3 cup dry beans = 1 cup cooked beans

½ cup dry beans = 1½ cups cooked beans

2/3 cup dry beans = 2 cups cooked beans

1 cup dry beans = 3 cups cooked beans

2 cups (1 pound) dry beans = 6 cups cooked beans

If you choose to use canned beans instead of cooking your own dried beans, make sure you select products that are labeled as "low sodium" or "no salt added".

Healthful Salad Dressings and Dips

Eat For Health is not a fat-free eating style because our bodies require healthy fats from whole foods, the way nature intended us to consume them. My eating style features creamy dressings and dips created with nuts, seeds and avocados. By eating this way, we receive the lignins, flavonoids, antioxidants, minerals, and other protective phytochemicals that come along in the package.

Salad dressings and dips usually start with oil and vinegar: the oil provides the fat and the vinegar provides the acidity. My salad dressings utilize whole foods as the fat sources: almond and cashews, other nuts and seeds, avocado, and tahini. These healthy fat sources are blended together in a high-powered blender or food processor with other healthy ingredients to create delicious creamy dressings and dips that you can feel good about indulging in. Always use raw nuts and seeds (or raw nut and seed butters) because the roasting process alters their beneficial fats. Commercially roasted nuts and seeds are often cooked in hydrogenated oils, adding trans fat to your diet.

Gourmet fruit-flavored vinegars are also used in many recipes, because they add unique and delicious flavors. Garlic, onions, fruit, Dijon mustard, and herbs and spices contribute additional character and interest.

Items from this chart can be combined to create new flavors while maintaining the nutritional quality of the dressings.

SALAD DRESSINGS – THE NUTRITARIAN WAY			
Flavor	**Fat**	**Acidity**	**Other**
Garlic	Almonds or Almond Butter	Balsamic Vinegar	Tofu
Onion	Cashews or Cashew Butter	Rice or Wine Vinegar	Soy, Hemp or Almond Milk
Fresh, Dried or Frozen Fruit	Sesame Seeds	Lemon Juice	100% Fruit or Vegetable Juice
Dijon Mustard	Pine Nuts	Flavored Vinegar	Low Sodium Tomato Sauce
Fresh or Dried Herbs	Pistachio or Other Nuts		
Spices (No Salt)	Hemp, Flax or Chia Seeds		
Dr. Fuhrman's VegiZest or MatoZest	Avocado		

Smoothies and Blended Salads

Blending raw vegetables with fruit is an efficient way to increase your nutrient absorption. All plants are composed of cells whose walls consist mainly of cellulose, a type of carbohydrate. Humans do not have the enzyme capable of breaking down cellulose, so we cannot utilize cellulose as an energy source. The only way we can break down these walls and release the most nutrients possible from the cells into the bloodstream is by thoroughly chewing.

When we chew a salad, we often don't do an efficient job of crushing every cell; about 70 to 90 percent of the cells are not broken open. As a result, most of the valuable nutrients contained within those cells never enter our bloodstream and are lost. This is one of the reasons why practicing the chewing exercises detailed in Chapter Five is so important. An even more efficient way to ensure you receive these nutrients is using a blender to puree raw, leafy greens.

A high-powered blender like the Vitamix brand is essential for making these smoothies and blended salads. The blending process aids your body in the work of breaking down and assimilating nutrients. It guarantees that a higher percentage of nutrients will be absorbed into your bloodstream. Making green smoothies or blended salads is a delicious and convenient way to pump up your consumption of greens.

Smoothies and blended salads can be made with endless combinations of vegetables, nuts, herbs, and condiments. They can be made to taste like gazpacho, creamy summer soups, a fruit shake, or a salad dressing. My typical green smoothie blends two ounces of lettuce, two ounces of spinach, a banana, some fresh or frozen fruit, a date, and half an avocado. You can add other greens, flavors and liquids according to your taste preferences. In the recipes provided in this book, we give you several options and encourage you to make your own combinations of everything from creamy cold vegetable soups to pudding-like desserts.

This chart will help you come up with new possibilities.

SMOOTHIES – THE NUTRITARIAN WAY			
Liquid (optional)	**Greens**	**Fruit** (Fresh or Frozen)	**Flavor/ Other**
Hemp, Almond or Soy Milk	Spinach	Berries– Blueberries, Strawberries, Raspberries	Dates or other Dried Fruit
Pomegranate Juice	Avocado	Cherries	Flax, Hemp or Chia Seeds
Orange Juice	Kale	Oranges	Goji Berries
Other 100% Fruit or Vegetable Juices	Lettuce	Banana	Non-alkalized, natural Cocoa Powder
Flavored Vinegars		Pineapple	Nuts
		Kiwi	Avocado
		Mango	Vanilla

Juicing

In addition to blending, I also recommend nutrient dense juices like my Mixed Vegetable Juice and the Raw Vegetable Cruciferous Juice. Recipes for these juices can be found in the recipe section of this book. With juicing, you retain many of the phytochemicals and other nutrients but lose other beneficial components like fiber and proteins.

Juicing should not replace the fruits or vegetables in your diet, but it is an effective way to boost your nutrient absorption because you can consume a lot of nutrients from raw green vegetables easily.

If you add a glass of freshly squeezed vegetable juice to your diet periodically or daily you can pump up your vegetable consumption easily and increase the availability and absorption of the anti-cancer phytochemical compounds.

If you have a digestive disorder, blending and juicing vegetables can be a great aid because you can increase your consumption of healing nutrients, even though your digestive capacity might be sub-par. Since eating a low-phytochemical, low-fiber diet goes against nature's design and causes most digestive disorders, eating a high-nutrient, vegetable-based diet often resolves digestive problems quickly. People suffering from irritable bowel syndrome, constipation, hemorrhoids, and reflux disease often see improvements after just a few weeks of juicing and eating blended salads. However, sometimes diets have to be modified for individual uniqueness or medical problems, such as ulcerative colitis or Crohn's disease, conditions that require fresh fruits and raw vegetables to be gradually introduced into the diet. In such cases, working with a knowledgeable physician may be helpful.

The high-nutrient availability of blended vegetables also helps normalize immune function in those suffering from asthma, allergies, and other immune system disorders. High-performance athletes or those interested in gaining weight can mix nuts and seeds into their blended vegetables. This combination supplies healthy sources of protein and fat in an efficiently absorbed, high-nutrient package.

Quick And Easy Meal Suggestions

This lifestyle does not have to be complicated. You may spend far less time in the kitchen than before. It is so easy to just shred some romaine lettuce and drizzle some tahini and lemon juice over it, heat up a tasty vegetable stew, or make a green smoothie. The nice outcome of eating this way is that even simple foods will taste better.

Don't forget to make creative use of leftovers. You do not need to cook every day. Plan to cook a healthful, nutrient-dense soup or stew two times a week. The leftovers can be used for lunch or dinners in the days that follow. The same can be done with dips and salad dressings. You do not have to use fancy recipes all the time. Simple foods are quick and easy and can work in this program too. Consider some of the options below to make your diet easier and more convenient.

Breakfast

Combine fresh fruit in season or even frozen fruit with raw nuts and seeds, or have a hot cereal, such as oatmeal, with cut up fruit on top. You could also make a quick smoothie with fruit and flax seeds, or have a hearty, whole-grain bread, like Alvarado Street, Manna Bread or Ezekiel brands, with trans-fat free spread or raw almond or cashew butter.

Lunch and Dinner

Your basic lunch should be a salad with a healthy dressing and a bowl of vegetable or bean soup that you made on the weekend. Make a quick salad from pre-mixed and pre-washed greens. Add chopped nuts, cut up fresh fruit or low-sodium canned beans and use a low-sodium dressing, fresh lemon, or balsamic or flavored vinegar. You can also eat raw vegetables and avocado with a low-sodium salsa or hummus dip or a low-sodium/low-fat store-bought dressing.

Try steaming some fresh broccoli, spinach or another green vegetable and adding fresh or dried herbs or spices. Baked sweet potato and corn on the cob with a trans-fat free spread or no-salt-added seasoning are great, easy options that are popular with children. A quick and tasty stir fry using the water sauté method learned in this chapter can be made from whatever fresh vegetables you have on hand. Defrosted frozen vegetables or fresh or frozen fruit are quick ways to round out a salad or leftover dish.

Another easy meal option is to stuff a 100% whole-grain pita bread or wrap with shredded romaine or other greens, tomato, dried tomatoes (pre-soaked in water), cucumber, bean sprouts, broccoli slaw, or cole slaw mix. You can add hummus, avocado, salsa, tahini, or nut butter. I often mash almond butter and tomato sauce together with Black Fig Vinegar and put it in the pita with tomatoes, avocado, and shredded lettuce.

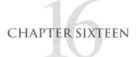

CHAPTER SIXTEEN

THREE LEVELS OF
SUPERIOR NUTRITION

I have organized my meal plans into three levels of superior nutrition. Based on your health needs and current dietary habits, you can choose between three different levels of superior nutrition, starting on Level 1, and working your way up to Level 3. I would like to see everyone reach at least Level 2, although for many people, Level 1 represents a significant improvement.

Over time, as your taste and food preferences change and you become more comfortable eating high-nutrient foods, consider moving to a higher level. Keep your focus on increasing your intake of disease-protective nutrients by eating natural whole foods.

Use my ANDI scores in Chapter 3 to help you choose more of the most nutrient-dense foods. When you eat foods with very high scores, you will be satisfied with fewer calories and will be less likely to overeat.

I have designed three levels, as an aid to direct people to the level of superior nutrition they need for their individual health conditions. This does not mean a person should not move to a higher level of excellence if they are comfortable doing so.

As you design your menus, keep in mind that the menus contained in this book provide approximately 1400 calories daily. For most people, this will result in moderate weight loss. If you do not need to lose weight, you can include some of the options listed at the bottom of each day's menu or include a more generous amount of raw nuts and seeds in your diet. Because this is not a calorie-counting diet, you do not need to worry about the size of your portions. Eat as much as you want without overeating. When you eat a micronutrient-rich diet, you naturally desire fewer calories. Everyone has different caloric needs, so you may require more or fewer calories than suggested in the menus. Eat when you are hungry. If you are not hungry, don't eat.

MENU GUIDELINES

Use the following high-nutrient guidelines as you design your individual menus.

FOR ALL LEVELS, INCLUDE DAILY:

1) A large salad
2) At least a half-cup serving of beans/legumes in soup, salad or a dish
3) At least 3 fresh fruits
4) At least one ounce of raw nuts and seeds
5) At least one large (double-size) serving of steamed green vegetables

AVOID:

1) barbecued, processed and cured meats and red meat
2) fried foods
3) full-fat dairy (cheese, ice cream, butter, whole milk or 2% milk) or trans fat (margarine)
4) soft drinks, sugar or artificial sweeteners
5) white flour products

Level 1 Guidelines

Level 1 is appropriate for a person who is healthy, thin, physically fit and exercises regularly. You should have no risk factors such as high blood pressure, high cholesterol or a family history of heart disease, stroke or cancer before the age of 75.

Most Americans do have risk factors or a family history of strokes, heart attacks and cancer, and most Americans are overweight. So most people should only see Level One as a temporary stage as they learn about high-nutrient eating and allow their taste buds to acclimate to higher levels of whole, natural plant foods.

Level 1 is designed to ease the emotional shock of making such profound dietary improvements. It enables people to revamp their diet at a level that is significant, but not overwhelming. Enjoy this new style of eating, allow your taste preferences to change with time and try some great recipes. You soon may decide to move on to a higher level. However, I still recommend that the majority of individuals make the commitment to jump right into the more nutrient dense Levels 2 or 3 because so many people are significantly overweight and have risk factors that need to be addressed immediately. People in desperate need of a health makeover need to start on Levels 2 or 3.

On Level 1, you eliminate fried foods and substitute fruit-based healthful desserts and whole grains for low-nutrient processed snack foods such as salty snacks, candy, ice cream and baked products. Whole grain products like old-fashioned oats, wild rice, brown rice, 100 percent whole grain bread and pasta with 100 percent whole grain or bean flour are used. Bread and pasta made with white flour are eliminated.

Your sodium intake will decrease as you begin to make these dietary changes. Processed foods and restaurant foods contribute 77 percent of the sodium people consume. Salt from the salt shaker provides 11% and sodium found naturally in food provides the remaining 12%.

You also eliminate foods like cheese and butter that are high in saturated fats. Your cooking techniques use only a minimal amount of oil. Most Americans consume over fifteen servings of animal products weekly. In Level 1, I recommend only four servings of animal products per week. These animal products are limited to fish, chicken, turkey, eggs or nonfat dairy products.

LEVEL 2 GUIDELINES

Level 2 builds on the positive changes described in Level 1. In Level 2, animal products are reduced to three servings weekly and vegetables and beans should start to make up an even larger portion of your total caloric intake. When you incorporate more and more nutrient-rich produce in your diet, you automatically increase your intake of antioxidants, phytochemicals, plant fibers, lignins, and plant sterols. You lower the glycemic index of your diet and the level of saturated fat, salt and other negative elements without having to think about it. Your ability to appreciate the natural flavors of unprocessed, whole foods will improve with time because you lose your dependence on salt and sugar. Add more beans and nuts to your diet to replace animal products. Try some of my high-nutrient dressing and dip recipes. They use heart healthy nuts and seeds to replace the oils found in traditional dressings and dips.

Level 2 is a good target diet for most people. If you want to lose weight, lower your cholesterol, lower your blood pressure, or just live a long healthy life, this is the level you should adopt.

LEVEL 3 GUIDELINES

If you suffer from serious medical conditions like diabetes, heart disease or autoimmune disease or just want to optimize the nutrient density of your diet to slow aging and maximize longevity, step up to Level 3. It is designed for those who want to reverse serious disease or for healthy people who want to push the envelope of human longevity.

Level 3 is the diet that I use in my medical practice when people have to reverse serious autoimmune diseases, (such as rheumatoid arthritis or lupus), or when someone has life-threatening heart disease (atherosclerosis). I prescribe it for diabetics who need to lower their blood sugars into the normal range, or to get rid of severe migraines. It delivers the highest level of nutrient density. It is also the level to choose if you have trouble losing weight, no matter what you do, and want to maximize your results.

Level 3 includes just two or fewer servings of animal products weekly and concentrates on high-nutrient density vegetables. Review my ANDI scores in Chapter Three to select the most nutrient-dense foods possible. Use green smoothies, fresh vegetable juices, healthful soups and lots of greens and raw vegetables to make every calorie count.

At this level, you should consume processed foods only rarely. Keep the use of refined fats and oils to a minimum. Nuts and seeds supply essential fats in a much healthier package, with significant health benefits.

OVERVIEW OF THE THREE LEVELS

	LEVEL 1	LEVEL 2	LEVEL 3
VEGETABLES raw & cooked 1 serving = 1-1/2 cups cooked or 2-5 cups raw	3-4 servings/day	4-6 servings/day	5-7 servings/day
FRUIT 1 serving = about 1-1/2 cups	3-5 servings/day	3-5 servings/day	3-5 servings/day
BEANS 1 serving = 1/2 to 1 cup	1-2 servings/day	1-2 servings/day	1-2 servings/day
NUTS & SEEDS 1 serving = 1 ounce or 1/4 cup	1-3 servings/day	1-3 servings/day	1-3 servings/day
	——— 1 serving/day if trying to lose weight ———		
WHOLE GRAIN PRODUCTS/POTATOES 1 serving = 1 slice or 1 cup	1-3 servings/day	1-3 servings/day	1-2 servings/day
ANIMAL PRODUCTS* 1 serving = 4 ounces	4 servings/week or less	3 servings/week or less	2 servings/week or less
SODIUM	1200 mg/day	1200 mg/day	1000 mg/day
FATS/OILS Substitutes include non-dairy spreads without trans or hydrogenated fats	1 tablespoon of olive oil or acceptable substitute/day	1 tablespoon of olive oil or acceptable substitute/day	1-2 tablespoons/week

* Animal Products include: white meat fowl, fish, eggs, low fat dairy. Absolutely no processed meats, cured meats, barbecued meat or full fat dairy.

Eat for Health In Practice

The most effective way to properly care for your health is to strive for superior nutrition. To do that, you must stay focused on the nutrient quality of the food you eat. However, this program doesn't demand perfection; nor does it mean that you will never eat meat again or that you will never have a slice of birthday cake. It means that your diet has been revamped so that high-nutrient fruits, vegetables, beans, and other foods make up the majority of your food intake, and that you have the knowledge and skills to come even closer to superior nutrition each day. The instances that you eat meat and cake will be fewer and you will find that, with time, those foods become less enjoyable. You may eventually choose not to eat them or other unhealthy foods because you have lost your desire and taste for them.

What you have read in this book has shown you that there is a whole body of nutritional information that has never been shared with the general public. Health professionals rarely use the power of lifestyle intervention and dietary modifications to help people suffering with serious medical problems. Instead, the emphasis is on intervention with pills, drugs, and surgeries. Commercial interests have dominated the nutritional messages shared with the public. The medical profession has become infatuated with technological advancements. This approach has not only failed to improve the general health of our nation, but has resulted in a dramatic explosion of the diseases of nutritional ignorance and excess. It has pushed health care spending through the roof without any improvement in healthy life expectancies . I hope every one of you who read this book can prove the strength of nutrition by achieving enhanced vigor and great health. Protecting yourself from a needless health tragedy is a gratifying experience that can bring satisfaction and pleasure to your life. Perhaps from your example, others will be encouraged to discover how rewarding it is to become a nutritarian.

Congratulations for seeking out the great rewards available to you, simply through changing your diet, when you "eat for health."

FOUR-WEEK MENU PLANS

Four weeks of menu plans and delicious recipes follow. Feel free to switch the foods or recipes around or use your own ideas and recipes as long as you follow the guidelines outlined in the previous chapters. Keep in mind that you do not necessarily have to make all these different dishes and recipes each week. Most of us make a soup or main dish and use the leftovers for lunch or even dinner the next day.

The following menus provide approximately 1400 calories daily. For most people, this will result in moderate weight loss. If you do not need to lose weight, you can also include some of the options listed at the bottom of each day's menu or include a more generous amount of raw nuts and seeds in your diet.

I consider the Level 2 menus to be a good starting point. You can use the tips and suggestions throughout this book to personalize your meals, adjusting the level of superior nutrition up or down to match your goals and health needs. If at a particular meal you want to move up or down a level, it is fine to do so.

Recipes printed in **BOLD TYPE** are included in
the recipe section that follows the menus.

WEEK ONE

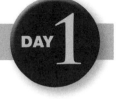

DAY 1

LEVEL 1	LEVEL 2	LEVEL 3

BREAKFAST··

whole grain bagel with trans-fat-free spread melon or other fresh fruit

Quick Banana Berry Breakfast To Go

Quick Banana Berry Breakfast To Go

LUNCH···

raw veggies

raw veggies

raw veggies

Tasty Hummus on a whole grain pita with mixed greens, tomato and chopped red pepper

grapes or other fresh fruit

Tasty Hummus on a whole grain pita with mixed greens, tomato and chopped red pepper

grapes or other fresh fruit

Apple Bok Choy Salad over mixed greens

grapes or other fresh fruit

DINNER···

mixed greens salad with assorted vegetables and **Tofu Ranch Dressing**

Golden Austrian Cauliflower Soup

Peach Sorbet

mixed greens salad with assorted vegetables and **Tofu Ranch Dressing**

Golden Austrian Cauliflower Soup

Peach Sorbet

mixed greens salad with assorted vegetables and **Tofu Ranch Dressing**

Golden Austrian Cauliflower Soup

Green Machine

Peach Sorbet

Options for higher calorie diets:
    LUNCH: add sliced avocado   **DINNER**: Acorn Squash Supreme

Menu items in **BOLD** indicate recipes in this book.

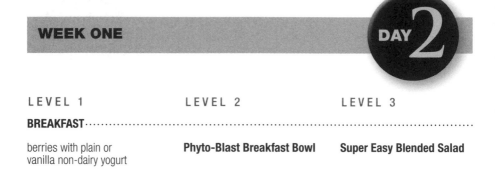

WEEK ONE

DAY 2

LEVEL 1	LEVEL 2	LEVEL 3

BREAKFAST···

berries with plain or vanilla non-dairy yogurt

Phyto-Blast Breakfast Bowl

Super Easy Blended Salad

LUNCH···

raw veggies with **Russian Fig Dressing**

raw veggies with **Russian Fig Dressing**

raw veggies with **Russian Fig Dressing**

Golden Austrian Cauliflower Soup (leftover)

Golden Austrian Cauliflower Soup (leftover)

Golden Austrian Cauliflower Soup (leftover)

pear or other fresh fruit

pear or other fresh fruit

pear or other fresh fruit

DINNER··

romaine salad with tomatoes and flavored vinegar

romaine salad with tomatoes and flavored vinegar

romaine salad with tomatoes and flavored vinegar

Creamed Forest Kale over Wild Rice (or brown rice) topped with 2 ounces of sliced chicken breast if desired

Creamed Forest Kale over Wild Rice (or brown rice) topped with 2 ounces of sliced chicken breast if desired

Creamed Forest Kale over Wild Rice

Options for higher calorie diets:
    DINNER: Russian Fig Dressing instead of flavored vinegar

DESSERT: Banana Oat Bars

Menu items in **BOLD** indicate recipes in this book.

WEEK ONE

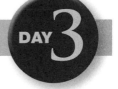

DAY **3**

LEVEL 1	LEVEL 2	LEVEL 3

BREAKFAST ··

whole grain cereal with fruit and soy, hemp or almond milk

Cinnamon Fruit Oatmeal

Cinnamon Fruit Oatmeal

Mixed Vegetable Juice

LUNCH ···

raw veggies with **Fresh Tomato Salsa**

Vegetable Bean Burrito with shredded lettuce and shredded non-dairy cheese

apple or other fresh fruit

raw veggies with **Fresh Tomato Salsa**

Vegetable Bean Burrito with shredded lettuce and shredded non-dairy cheese

apple or other fresh fruit

raw veggies with **Fresh Tomato Salsa**

Southern Style Mixed Greens

apple or other fresh fruit

DINNER ··

mixed greens and arugula salad with choice of *Eat for Health* dressings

Broccoli Lentil Soup

mixed greens and arugula salad with choice of *Eat for Health* dressings

Broccoli Lentil Soup

mixed greens and arugula salad with choice of *Eat for Health* dressings

Broccoli Lentil Soup

Swiss Chard with Garlic and Lemon

Options for higher calorie diets:
 LUNCH: add sliced avocado

DINNER: top salad with pine nuts or pumpkin seeds

Menu items in **BOLD** indicate recipes in this book.

WEEK ONE

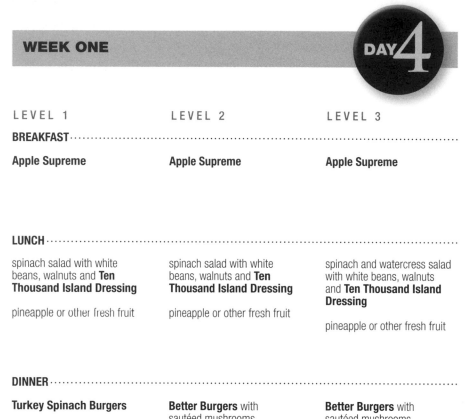

DAY 4

LEVEL 1	LEVEL 2	LEVEL 3

BREAKFAST

Apple Supreme

Apple Supreme

Apple Supreme

LUNCH

spinach salad with white beans, walnuts and **Ten Thousand Island Dressing**

pineapple or other fresh fruit

spinach salad with white beans, walnuts and **Ten Thousand Island Dressing**

pineapple or other fresh fruit

spinach and watercress salad with white beans, walnuts and **Ten Thousand Island Dressing**

pineapple or other fresh fruit

DINNER

Turkey Spinach Burgers

Sweet Potato Fires

strawberries dusted with cocoa powder

Better Burgers with sautéed mushrooms, chopped red onion on a 100% whole grain bun

Triple Treat Cabbage Salad

strawberries dusted with cocoa powder

Better Burgers with sautéed mushrooms, chopped red onion

Great Greens

Triple Treat Cabbage Salad

strawberries dusted with cocoa powder

Options for higher calorie diets:
    LUNCH: Roasted Vegetable Pizza   **DESSERT: Chocolate Dip for strawberries**

Menu items in **BOLD** indicate recipes in this book.

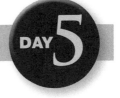

WEEK ONE

DAY 5

LEVEL 1	LEVEL 2	LEVEL 3

BREAKFAST

| Blueberry Orange Smoothie | Eat Your Greens Fruit Smoothie | Eat Your Greens Fruit Smoothie |

LUNCH

| **Vegetable Garbanzo Wraps** | **Vegetable Garbanzo Wraps** | steamed Vegetables with **Sesame Ginger Sauce** |
| berries or other fresh fruit | berries or other fresh fruit | berries or other fresh fruit |

DINNER

mixed greens salad with assorted vegetables and **Almond Balsamic Vinaigrette**	mixed greens salad with assorted vegetables and **Almond Balsamic Vinaigrette**	mixed greens salad with assorted vegetables and **Almond Balsamic Vinaigrette**
Chunky Sweet Potato Stew	**Tuscan Greens and Beans Soup**	**Tuscan Greens and Beans Soup**
Blueberry Banana Cobbler	**Blueberry Banana Cobbler**	**Blueberry Banana Cobbler**

Options for higher calorie diets:
   BREAKFAST: add banana with raw cashew or almond butter

LUNCH: add unsulfured dried figs

> Menu items in **BOLD** indicate recipes in this book.

WEEK ONE

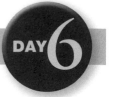

DAY 6

LEVEL 1	LEVEL 2	LEVEL 3

BREAKFAST

whole grain cereal with fruit and soy, hemp or almond milk

Phyto-Blast Breakfast Bowl

Dr. Fuhrman's Fruit, Nut and Veggie Breakfast

LUNCH

Chunky Sweet Potato Stew (leftover)

melon or other fresh fruit

Tuscan Greens & Beans Soup (leftover)

melon or other fresh fruit

Tuscan Greens & Beans Soup (leftover)

melon or other fresh fruit

DINNER

spinach salad with lightly sautéed mushrooms and **Orange Sesame Dressing**

Salmon and Vegetables in a Packet
(*vegan option:* substitute extra firm tofu for salmon)

brown & wild rice

spinach salad with lightly sautéed mushrooms and **Orange Sesame Dressing**

Salmon and Vegetables in a Packet
(*vegan option:* substitute extra firm tofu for salmon)

brown & wild rice

spinach salad with lightly sautéed mushrooms and **Orange Sesame Dressing**

Salmon and Vegetables in a Packet
(*vegan option:* substitute extra firm tofu for salmon)

Braised Bok Choy

Options for higher calorie diets:
  DESSERT: Banana Walnut Ice Cream

Menu items in **BOLD** indicate recipes in this book.

WEEK ONE

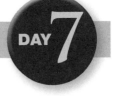

DAY 7

LEVEL 1

BREAKFAST··

**Scrambled Veggies
and Eggs**
(*vegan option:* **Deluxe Tofu
Scramble**)

mango or other fresh fruit

LEVEL 2

**Scrambled Veggies
and Eggs**
(*vegan option:* **Deluxe Tofu
Scramble**)

mango or other fresh fruit

LEVEL 3

Vegetable Omelet
(*vegan option:* **Quinoa
Breakfast**)

High Cruciferous Juice

LUNCH··

**Portobello Red Pepper
Sandwich**

berries or other fresh fruit

**Portobello Red Pepper
Sandwich**

berries or other fresh fruit

**Portobello Red Pepper
Sandwich**

berries or other fresh fruit

DINNER···

romaine salad with
Cashew Caesar Dressing

**Pasta with Roasted
Vegetables**

romaine salad with
Cashew Caesar Dressing

**Spaghetti Squash
Primavera**

romaine and arugula salad
with **Cashew Caesar
Dressing**

**Spaghetti Squash
Primavera**

Options for higher calorie diets:
   BREAKFAST: whole grain toast with 100%
   fruit spread

DESSERT: Summer Fruit Pie

Menu items in **BOLD** indicate recipes in this book.

WEEK TWO

DAY 1

LEVEL 1 | LEVEL 2 | LEVEL 3

BREAKFAST

Apple Pie Smoothie

Chocolate Smoothie

Chocolate Smoothie

LUNCH

mixed greens salad with assorted vegetables, walnuts and purchased low-fat, low-sodium dressing

orange or other fresh fruit

Citrus Salad with Orange Peanut Dressing

Citrus Salad with Orange Peanut Dressing

DINNER

Baked Garlic Pita Chips with **Simple Guacamole**

Easy Three Bean Vegetable Chili

quinoa

raw vegetables with **Simple Guacamole**

Easy Three Bean Vegetable Chili

quinoa

raw vegetables with **Simple Guacamole**

Easy Three Bean Vegetable Chili

Supreme Kale

Options for higher calorie diets:
BREAKFAST: add banana with raw cashew or almond butter

DINNER: add cooked sweet potato or butternut squash to chili

Menu items in **BOLD** indicate recipes in this book.

WEEK TWO

DAY 2

LEVEL 1

BREAKFAST

Cinnamon Fruit Oatmeal

100% fruit juice

LEVEL 2

Cinnamon Fruit Oatmeal

100% fruit juice

LEVEL 3

Cinnamon Fruit Oatmeal

Mixed Vegetable Juice

LUNCH

edamame with no-salt seasoning

Easy Bean & Vegetable Chili (leftover)

kiwi or other fresh fruit

edamame with no-salt seasoning

Easy Bean & Vegetable Chili (leftover)

kiwi or other fresh fruit

edamame with no-salt seasoning

Easy Bean & Vegetable Chili (leftover)

kiwi or other fresh fruit

DINNER

mixed greens with shredded cabbage and **Almond Balsamic Vinaigrette**

Eggplant Roll Ups

whole grain pasta

Apple Surprise

mixed greens with shredded cabbage and **Almond Balsamic Vinaigrette**

Eggplant Roll Ups

steamed broccoli

Apple Surprise

mixed greens with shredded cabbage and **Almond Balsamic Vinaigrette**

Eggplant Roll Ups

Spinach and Brussels Sprouts Delight

Apple Surprise

Options for higher calorie diets:
DESSERT: Serve **Apple Surprise** with **Frozen Banana Fluff**

Menu items in **BOLD** indicate recipes in this book.

WEEK TWO

DAY 3

LEVEL 1	LEVEL 2	LEVEL 3

BREAKFAST

whole grain cereal with fruit and soy, hemp or almond milk

Tropical Fruit Salad with ground hemp or chia seeds

Tropical Fruit Salad with ground hemp or chia seeds over shredded romaine

LUNCH

Herbed White Bean Hummus on a whole grain pita with romaine, tomato and shredded carrots

watermelon or other fresh fruit

Herbed White Bean Hummus on a whole grain pita with romaine, tomato and shredded carrots

watermelon or other fresh fruit

Black Bean Lettuce Bundles

watermelon or other fresh fruit

DINNER

mixed greens salad with chopped red onion and purchased low-fat, low-sodium dressing

Black Forest Cream of Mushroom Soup

Very Berry Sorbet

mixed greens salad with chopped red onion and **Tofu Ranch Dressing**

Black Forest Cream of Mushroom Soup

Very Berry Sorbet

mixed greens and watercress salad with chopped red onion and **Tofu Ranch Dressing**

Black Forest Cream of Mushroom Soup

Very Berry Sorbet

Options for higher calorie diets:
LUNCH: add sliced avocado

DINNER: add **Sweet Potato Fries**

Menu items in **BOLD** indicate recipes in this book.

WEEK TWO

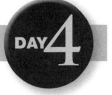

DAY 4

LEVEL 1	LEVEL 2	LEVEL 3

BREAKFAST

Phyto Blast Breakfast Bowl

Blended Mango Salad

Blended Mango Salad

LUNCH

Speedy Vegetable Wrap

berries or other fresh fruit

Black Forest Cream of Mushroom Soup (loftovor)

berries or other fresh fruit

Black Forest Cream of Mushroom Soup (leftover)

berries or other fresh fruit

DINNER

Walnut Pear Green Salad

Turkey Vegetable Meatloaf
(*vegan option:* **Garden Stuffed Vegetables**)

baked potato with trans-free spread and no-salt seasoning

Walnut Pear Green Salad

Turkey Vegetable Meatloaf
(*vegan option:* **Garden Stuffed Vegetables**)

California Creamed Kale

mixed greens salad with
Blueberry Pomegranate Dressing

Garden Stuffed Vegetables

California Creamed Kale

Options for higher calorie diets:
 BREAKFAST: add **Banana Cashew Lettuce Wrap**

LUNCH: add unsulfured dried apricots or figs

Menu items in **BOLD** indicate recipes in this book.

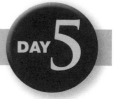

WEEK TWO

DAY 5

LEVEL 1	LEVEL 2	LEVEL 3

BREAKFAST··

Quick Banana
Breakfast To Go

Quick Banana
Breakfast To Go

Quick Banana
Breakfast To Go

High Cruciferous Juice

LUNCH··

Italian Stuffer with 2 ounces
of baked turkey or chicken if
desired

cherries or other fresh fruit

Italian Stuffer

cherries or other fresh fruit

Collard Dijon Wrap Ups

cherries or other fresh fruit

DINNER···

romaine and mixed greens
salad with assorted vegetables
and **Russian Fig Dressing**

No-Meat Balls with low
sodium pasta sauce

whole grain pasta

Garlicky Zucchini

romaine and mixed greens
salad with assorted vegetables
and **Russian Fig Dressing**

No-Meat Balls with low
sodium pasta sauce

baked spaghetti squash

Garlicky Zucchini

romaine and mixed greens
salad with assorted vegetables
and **Russian Fig Dressing**

No-Meat Balls with low
sodium pasta sauce

baked spaghetti squash

**Swiss Chard with
Garlic and Lemon**

Options for higher calorie diets:
DESSERT: **Chocolate Cherry Sorbet**

Menu items in **BOLD** indicate recipes in this book.

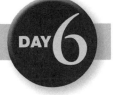

WEEK TWO

DAY 6

LEVEL 1

BREAKFAST

whole grain toast with trans-fat free spread

LEVEL 2

Antioxidant-Rich Bars

LEVEL 3

Antioxidant-Rich Bars

LUNCH

Roasted Vegetable Pizza

orange or other fresh fruit

Roasted Vegetable Pizza

orange or other fresh fruit

Greens and Berries Salad with Cashew Currant Dressing

DINNER

spinach salad with **Ginger Almond Dressing**

Creole Chicken with Spinach
(*vegan option:* **Thai Vegetable Curry**)

spinach salad with **Ginger Almond Dressing**

Creole Chicken with Spinach
(*vegan option:* **Thai Vegetable Curry**)

spinach salad with **Ginger Almond Dressing**

Thai Vegetable Curry

Options for higher calorie diets:
  BREAKFAST: soy, hemp or almond milk

DESSERT: Bluevado Pie

Menu items in **BOLD** indicate recipes in this book.

WEEK TWO

DAY 7

LEVEL 1	LEVEL 2	LEVEL 3
BREAKFAST		
Vegetable Omelet (*vegan option:* **Quinoa Breakfast**)	**Vegetable Omelet** (*vegan option:* **Quinoa Breakfast**)	Quinoa Breakfast
		High Cruciferious Juice
100% fruit juice	100% fruit juice	
LUNCH		
Black Bean Mango Salad	Black Bean Mango Salad	Black Bean Mango Salad
DINNER		
raw Veggies with **Tasty Hummus**	raw Veggies with **Tasty Hummus**	**Triple Treat Cabbage Salald**
Pasta with Roasted Vegetables	**Vegetable Shepherd's Pie**	**Vegetable Shepherd's Pie**

Options for higher calorie diets:
   LUNCH: Top mango salad with pumpkin seeds

DESSERT: Blueberry Banana Cobbler

Menu items in **BOLD** indicate recipes in this book.

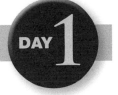

WEEK THREE

DAY 1

LEVEL 1	LEVEL 2	LEVEL 3

BREAKFAST

LEVEL 1	LEVEL 2	LEVEL 3
whole grain cereal with fruit and soy, hemp or almond milk	**Banana Cashew Lettuce Wrap**	**Eat Your Greens Fruit Smoothie**

LUNCH

LEVEL 1	LEVEL 2	LEVEL 3
Tasty Hummus with mixed greens, tomato and chopped red onion on sprouted wheat bread	**Greek Chickpea Salad**	**Greek Chickpea Salad**
melon or other fresh fruit	melon or other fresh fruit	melon or other fresh fruit

DINNER

LEVEL 1	LEVEL 2	LEVEL 3
mixed greens salad with **Blueberry Pomegranate Dressing**	mixed greens salad with **Blueberry Pomegranate Dressing**	mixed greens and watercress salad with **Blueberry Pomegranate Dressing**
Dr. Fuhrman's Famous Anti-Cancer Soup	**Dr. Fuhrman's Famous Anti-Cancer Soup**	**Dr. Fuhrman's Famous Anti-Cancer Soup**
Red Velvet Sorbet	**Red Velvet Sorbet**	**Red Velvet Sorbet**

Options for higher calorie diets:
DINNER: add dried blueberries, raisins
or walnuts to salad

Menu items in **BOLD** indicate recipes in this book.

WEEK THREE

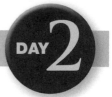

DAY 2

LEVEL 1	LEVEL 2	LEVEL 3

BREAKFAST

Wild Blueberry Hot Breakfast	**Pomegranate Muesli**	**Pomegranate Muesli**
		Refreshing Sunrise Juice

LUNCH

red pepper and carrot sticks with **Spicy Bean Dip**	red pepper and carrot sticks with **Spicy Bean Dip**	red pepper and carrot sticks with **Spicy Bean Dip**
Dr. Fuhrman's Anti-Cancer Soup (leftover)	**Dr. Fuhrman's Anti-Cancer Soup** (leftover)	**Dr. Fuhrman's Anti-Cancer Soup** (leftover)
apple or other fresh fruit	apple or other fresh fruit	apple or other fresh fruit

DINNER

Turkey Vegetable Meatloaf	**Artichoke Lentil Loaf**	**Artichoke Lentil Loaf**
Mushroom Stroganoff	**Mushroom Stroganoff**	**Mushroom Stroganoff**
baked sweet potato	steamed asparagus	**Supreme Kale**

Options for higher calorie diets:
  LUNCH: apple with raw cashew
  or almond butter

Menu items in **BOLD** indicate recipes in this book.

WEEK THREE

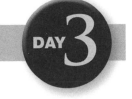

DAY 3

LEVEL 1	LEVEL 2	LEVEL 3

BREAKFAST

Tropical Mint Smoothie   **Antioxidant-Rich Smoothie**   **Antioxidant-Rich Smoothie**

LUNCH

Spinach and Garbanzo Bean Salad with Lemon Fig Dressing	**Spinach and Garbanzo Bean Salad with Lemon Fig Dressing**	**Broccoli and Spinach Microsalad**
grapes or other fresh fruit	grapes or other fresh fruit	grapes or other fresh fruit

DINNER

Apple Cinnamon Butternut Squash Soup	**Apple Cinnamon Butternut Squash Soup**	**Apple Cinnamon Butternut Squash Soup**
Southwest Vegetable Stew	**Quick Vegetable Bean Medley**	**Quick Vegetable Bean Medley**

Options for higher calorie diets:
   LUNCH: top salad with currants or raisins   **DINNER:** add brown or wild rice

Menu items in **BOLD** indicate recipes in this book.

WEEK THREE

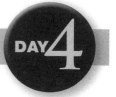

DAY 4

LEVEL 1	LEVEL 2	LEVEL 3

BREAKFAST ···

fresh fruit and sunflower seeds with non-dairy plain or vanilla yogurt	**Special Oatmeal**	**Special Oatmeal**

LUNCH ···

salad with mixed greens, assorted vegetables, beans and **Dijon Pistachio Dressing**	salad with mixed greens, assorted vegetables, beans and **Dijon Pistachio Dressing**	salad with mixed greens, assorted vegetables, beans and **Dijon Pistachio Dressing**
watermelon or other fresh fruit	watermelon or other fresh fruit	watermelon or other fresh fruit

DINNER ···

Baked Garlic Pita Chips	raw veggies	raw veggies
Fresh Tomato Salsa	**Fresh Tomato Salsa**	**Fresh Tomato Salsa**
Bean Enchiladas	**Bean Enchiladas**	**Mediterranean Bean and Kale Sauté**
Strawberry Pineapple Sorbet	**Strawberry Pineapple Sorbet**	**Strawberry Pineapple Sorbet**

Options for higher calorie diets:
BREAKFAST: add 100% fruit juice or low sodium vegetable juice

DINNER: serve pita chips or veggies with **Simple Guacamole**

Menu items in **BOLD** indicate recipes in this book.

WEEK THREE

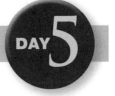

DAY 5

LEVEL 1

BREAKFAST ·

Tropcial Fruit Salad

LEVEL 2

Chocolate Cherry Smoothie

LEVEL 3

Chocolate Cherry Smoothie

LUNCH ·

whole grain wrap with turkey or hummus, lettuce, tomato and avocado

berries or other fresh fruit

Portobello Wraps with Watercress Salsa

berries or other fresh fruit

Portobello Wraps with Watercress Salsa

berries or other fresh fruit

DINNER ·

romaine salad with red pepper and **Banana Walnut Dressing**

Creamy Zucchini Soup

romaine salad with red pepper and **Banana Walnut Dressing**

Creamy Zucchini Soup

romaine salad with red pepper and **Banana Walnut Dressing**

Creamy Cruciferous Curry

Options for higher calorie diets:
DESSERT: Wild Apple Crunch

Menu items in **BOLD** indicate recipes in this book.

WEEK THREE

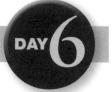

DAY 6

LEVEL 1	LEVEL 2	LEVEL 3

BREAKFAST

Garden Eggs and Tofu with Salsa
(*vegan option:* **Deluxe Tofu Scramble**)

Garden Eggs and Tofu with Salsa
(*vegan option:* **Deluxe Tofu Scramble**)

Garden Eggs and Tofu with Salsa
(*vegan option:* **Deluxe Tofu Scramble**)

Mixed Vegetable Juice

LUNCH

Triple Treat Cabbage Salad

Creamy Zucchini Soup
(leftover)

Triple Treat Cabbage Salad

Creamy Zucchini Soup
(leftover)

Triple Treat Cabbage Salad

Creamy Cruciferous Curry
(leftover)

DINNER

Kale Pesto over Pasta and Beans

Poached Pears with Raspberry Sauce

No Pasta Vegetable Lasagna

Poached Pears with Raspberry Sauce

No Pasta Vegetable Lasagna

Poached Pears with Raspberry Sauce

Options for higher calorie diets:
LUNCH: add apple with raw cashew or almond butter

DINNER: top entrée with pine nuts

Menu items in **BOLD** indicate recipes in this book.

WEEK THREE

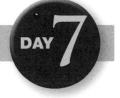

DAY 7

LEVEL 1   LEVEL 2   LEVEL 3

BREAKFAST

LEVEL 1	LEVEL 2	LEVEL 3
100% whole grain bagel with trans-free spread	**Quinoa Breakfast**	**Quinoa Breakfast**
berries or other fresh fruit		

LUNCH

LEVEL 1	LEVEL 2	LEVEL 3
raw veggies	**Super Slaw**	**Super Slaw**
Pita stuffed with Seasoned Greens	**Pita stuffed with Seasoned Greens**	**French Minted Pea Soup**
orange or other fresh fruit	orange or other fresh fruit	orange or other fresh fruit

DINNER

LEVEL 1	LEVEL 2	LEVEL 3
romalne and tomato salad with choice of **Eat for Health Dressings**	romaine and tomato salad with choice of **Eat for Health Dressings**	romaine, watercress and tomato salad with choice of **Eat for Health Dressings**
Asian Vegetable Stir Fry with small pieces of chicken or shrimp if desired	**Asian Vegetable Stir Fry** with small pieces of chicken or shrimp if desired	**Asian Vegetable Stir Fry** with small pieces of chicken or shrimp if desired
fresh strawberries	fresh strawberries	fresh strawberries

Options for higher calorie diets:
DESSERT: serve **Chocolate Dip** with
fresh strawberries

Menu items in **BOLD** indicate recipes in this book.

WEEK FOUR

DAY 1

LEVEL 1	LEVEL 2	LEVEL 3

BREAKFAST

LEVEL 1	LEVEL 2	LEVEL 3
Oatmeal with Fruit Compote	**Oatmeal with Fruit Compote**	**Oatmeal with Fruit Compote**
100% fruit juice	100% fruit juice	**Mixed Vegetable Juice**

LUNCH

LEVEL 1	LEVEL 2	LEVEL 3
Black Bean Lettuce Bundles	**Black Bean Lettuce Bundles**	**Black Bean Lettuce Bundles**
Dijon Vinaigrette Asparagus	**Dijon Vinaigrette Asparagus**	**Dijon Vinaigrette Asparagus**
pear or other fresh fruit	pear or other fresh fruit	pear or other fresh fruit

DINNER

LEVEL 1	LEVEL 2	LEVEL 3
Baked Garlic Pita Chips with **Grandma Tillie's Eggplant Dip**	raw veggies with **Grandma Tillie's Eggplant Dip**	raw veggies with **Grandma Tillie's Eggplant Dip**
Tomato Bisque Soup	**Tomato Bisque Soup**	**High Cruciferous Vegetable Stew**

Options for higher calorie diets:
   LUNCH: add sprouted grain bread

DESSERT: Banana Walnut Ice Cream

Menu items in **BOLD** indicate recipes in this book.

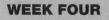

WEEK FOUR

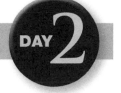
DAY 2

LEVEL 1   LEVEL 2   LEVEL 3

BREAKFAST

Vegetable Omelet
(*vegan option:* **Deluxe Tofu Scramble**)

Vegetable Omelet
(*vegan option:* **Deluxe Tofu Scramble**)

Vegetable Omelet
(*vegan option:* **Deluxe Tofu Scramble**)

LUNCH

mixed greens salad with assorted vegetables and flavored vinegar

mixed greens salad with assorted vegetables and flavored vinegar

mixed greens salad with assorted vegetables and flavored vinegar

Tomato Bisque Soup
(leftover)

Tomato Bisque Soup
(leftover)

High Cruciferous Vegetable Stew (leftover)

cherries or other fresh fruit

cherries or other fresh fruit

cherries or other fresh fruit

DINNER

Cuban Black Beans
with brown rice

Swiss Chard and Sweet Potato Gratin

Swiss Chard and Sweet Potato Gratin

Broccoli Fra Diavlo

Broccoli Fra Diavlo

Broccoli Fra Diavlo

Dr. Fuhrman's Banana Oat Cookies

Dr. Fuhrman's Banana Oat Cookies

Dr. Fuhrman's Banana Oat Cookies

Options for higher calorie diets:
LUNCH: Substitute Choice of *Eat for Health* **Dressings** for flavored vinegar and top salad with chopped nuts or seeds

Menu items in **BOLD** indicate recipes in this book.

WEEK FOUR

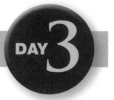

DAY 3

LEVEL 1	LEVEL 2	LEVEL 3

BREAKFAST

mixed berries topped with **Berry "Yogurt"**	mixed berries topped with **Berry "Yogurt"**	mixed berries topped with **Berry "Yogurt"**

LUNCH

turkey or **Black Bean Hummus** on a whole grain wrap with shredded lettuce, tomato and avocado grapes or other fresh fruit	**Quinoa Bean Salad** on a bed of mixed greens grapes or other fresh fruit	**Quinoa Bean Salad** on a bed of mixed greens grapes or other fresh fruit

DINNER

Pistachio Crusted Tempeh with Balsamic and Shiitake Mushrooms **Lemon Zest Spinach** **Jenna's Peach Freeze**	**Pistachio Crusted Tempeh with Balsamic and Shiitake Mushrooms** **Lemon Zest Spinach** **Jenna's Peach Freeze**	**Pistachio Crusted Tempeh with Balsamic and Shiitake Mushrooms** **Spinach and Brussels Sprouts Delight** **Jenna's Peach Freeze**

Options for higher calorie diets:
   BREAKFAST OR DESSERT: Orange Goji Bars

Menu items in **BOLD** indicate recipes in this book.

WEEK FOUR

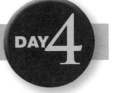

DAY 4

LEVEL 1

LEVEL 2

LEVEL 3

BREAKFAST

Apple Pie Smoothie

Antioxidant-Rich Smoothie

Antioxidant-Rich Smoothie

LUNCH

romaine and spinach salad
with **Cashew Caesar
Dressing**

Roasted Vegetable Pizza

Melon or other fresh fruit

romalne and spinach salad
with **Cashew Caesar
Dressing**

Roasted Vegetable Pizza

Melon or other fresh fruit

romaine and spinach salad
with **Cashew Caesar
Dressing**

steamed vegetables with low
sodium tomato sauce

Melon or other fresh fruit

DINNER

**Spinach Stuffed
Mushrooms**

**Quick and Creamy
Vegetable Bean Soup**

**Spinach Stuffed
Mushrooms**

**Quick and Creamy
Vegetable Bean Soup**

**Spinach Stuffed
Mushrooms**

**Quick and Creamy
Vegetable Bean Soup**

Options for higher calorie diets:
BREAKFAST: add unsulfured dried figs
or apricots

DINNER: add baked sweet potato

Menu items in **BOLD** indicate recipes in this book.

WEEK FOUR

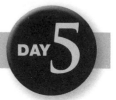

DAY 5

LEVEL 1	LEVEL 2	LEVEL 3

BREAKFAST

whole grain cereal with fruit and soy, hemp or almond milk

Special Oatmeal

Special Oatmeal

LUNCH

endive spears with **Black Bean Hummus**

Quick and Creamy Vegetable Bean Soup (leftover)

pineapple or other fresh fruit

endive spears with **Black Bean Hummus**

Quick and Creamy Vegetable Bean Soup (leftover)

pineapple or other fresh fruit

endive spears with **Black Bean Hummus**

Quick and Creamy Vegetable Bean Soup (leftover)

pineapple or other fresh fruit

DINNER

Turkey Vegetable Meatloaf (*vegan option:* **Thanksgiving Non-Meat Loaf**)

Cauliflower Spinach Mashed "Potatoes"

steamed green beans

Thanksgiving Non-Meat Loaf

Cauliflower Spinach Mashed "Potatoes"

steamed green beans

Thanksgiving Non-Meat Loaf

Cauliflower Spinach Mashed "Potatoes"

Orange Sesame Kale

Options for higher calorie diets:
DESSERT: Dr. Fuhrman's Banana Nut Cookies

Menu items in **BOLD** indicate recipes in this book.

WEEK FOUR

DAY **6**

LEVEL 1

LEVEL 2

LEVEL 3

BREAKFAST ·

Phyto Blast Breakfast Bowl

Phyto Blast Breakfast Bowl

Phyto Blast Breakfast Bowl

LUNCH ·

whole grain pita stuffed with greens, lettuce, broccoli slaw and **Zesty Avocado Dressing**

mango or other fresh fruit

mixed greens, spinach, assorted vegetables and black bean salad with **Zesty Avocado Dressing**

mango or other fresh fruit

Braised Kale and Squash with Pumpkin Seeds

mango or other fresh fruit

DINNER ·

Fresh Beet Hummus with whole grain pita triangles

Mediterranean Fish Stew (*vegan option:* **Spaghetti Squash Primavera**)

brown rice

Fresh Beet Hummus with raw vegetables

Mediterranean Fish Stew (*vegan option:* **Spaghetti Squash Primavera**)

Herbed Barley and Lentils

Fresh Beet Hummus with raw vegetables

Mediterranean Fish Stew (*vegan option:* **Spaghetti Squash Primavera**)

Herbed Barley and Lentils with steamed broccoli

Options for higher calorie diets:
BREAKFAST: add **Banana Cashew Lettuce Wrap**

DESSERT: choice of *Eat for Health* desserts

Menu items in **BOLD** indicate recipes in this book.

WEEK FOUR

DAY 7

LEVEL 1 | LEVEL 2 | LEVEL 3

BREAKFAST ....

Quick Banana Berry Breakfast To Go

Quick Banana Berry Breakfast To Go

Quick Banana Berry Breakfast To Go

LUNCH ....

Bean Enchiladas with **Fresh Tomato Salsa**

papaya or other fresh fruit

Bean Enchiladas with **Fresh Tomato Salsa**

papaya or other fresh fruit

Cremini Ratatouille

papaya or other fresh fruit

DINNER ....

Steamed Artichoke dipped in **Cashew Caesar Dressing**

Roasted Vegetable Pizza

Healthy Chocolate Cake

Steamed Artichoke dipped in **Cashew Caesar Dressing**

Vegetable Tagine

brown and wild rice

Healthy Chocolate Cake

Steamed Artichoke dipped in **Cashew Caesar Dressing**

Vegetable Tagine

steamed cauliflower

brown and wild rice

Healthy Chocolate Cake

Options for higher calorie diets:
   BREAKFAST: add 100% fruit juice   **LUNCH**: add sliced avocado

Menu items in **BOLD** indicate recipes in this book.

Eat for Health
Recipe Index

NON-VEGAN DISHES

DESSERTS

RECIPES

RECIPES

Some of the recipes in this book contain Dr. Fuhrman's Black Fig Vinegar, Dr. Fuhrman's Blood Orange Vinegar, Dr. Fuhrman's Riesling Reserve Vinegar, Dr. Fuhrman's Blueberry Vinegar, Dr. Fuhrman's Spicy Pecan Vinegar, Dr. Fuhrman's D'Anjou Pear Vinegar, Dr. Fuhrman's VegiZest and/or Dr. Fuhrman's MatoZest. I include these premixed options, available at DrFuhrman.com or fine health food stores, for your convenience; however, the recipes can be made without them. If you use one of the alternate ingredients that I suggest in a recipe, start with a small amount and add more according to your own taste, as the intensity of spice products can differ markedly from brand to brand.

SMOOTHIES, BLENDED SALADS AND JUICES

—SMOOTHIES AND BLENDED SALADS—

APPLE PIE SMOOTHIE

Serves: 2

INGREDIENTS

2 medium apples*

3 dates, pitted

1/4 cup walnuts

1/4 cup raisins

1 teaspoon cinnamon

1/4 teaspoon vanilla

1 tablespoon ground chia seeds

1 1/2 cups unsweetened soy, hemp or almond milk

DIRECTIONS

Blend all ingredients in a high powered blender until smooth and creamy.

* No need to peel apple if organic

PER SERVING: CALORIES 373; PROTEIN 15g; CARBOHYDRATES 56g; TOTAL FAT 14.9g; SATURATED FAT 1.5g; SODIUM 104mg; FIBER 9.9g; BETA-CAROTENE 700ug; VITAMIN C 7mg; CALCIUM 128mg; IRON 3.7mg; FOLATE 54ug; MAGNESIUM 100mg; ZINC 1.6mg; SELENIUM 10.7ug

Antioxidant-Rich Smoothie

Serves: 2

INGREDIENTS

- 4 cups baby spinach
- 4 cups romaine lettuce
- 1 cup pomegranate juice
- 1 cup frozen blueberries
- 1 cup frozen strawberries
- 4 dates, pitted
- 2 tablespoons ground chia seeds
- 1/2 ripe avocado, peeled and pitted

DIRECTIONS

Blend all ingredients together in a high powered blender until smooth and creamy.

PER SERVING: CALORIES 358; PROTEIN 7g; CARBOHYDRATES 63g; TOTAL FAT 11.8g; SATURATED FAT 1.9g; SODIUM 68mg; FIBER 14.8g; BETA-CAROTENE 7361ug; VITAMIN C 90mg; CALCIUM 146mg; IRON 4.1mg; FOLATE 323ug; MAGNESIUM 128mg; ZINC 1.4mg; SELENIUM 3.9ug

BLENDED MANGO SALAD

Serves: 2

INGREDIENTS

2 ripe mangos

1 cup chopped spinach

4 cups chopped romaine lettuce

1/4 cup unsweetened soy, hemp or almond milk

DIRECTIONS

Peel and chop mangos and place in food processor or high powered blender.

Add spinach and half the lettuce. Blend until well combined. Add the milk and remaining lettuce. Blend until creamy.

PER SERVING: CALORIES 105; PROTEIN 4g; CARBOHYDRATES 22g; TOTAL FAT 1.4g; SATURATED FAT 0.2g; SODIUM 24mg; FIBER 4.8g; BETA-CAROTENE 5207ug; VITAMIN C 60mg; CALCIUM 67mg; IRON 1.9mg; FOLATE 203ug; MAGNESIUM 44mg; ZINC 0.5mg; SELENIUM 1.2ug

BLUEBERRY ORANGE SMOOTHIE

Serves: 2

INGREDIENTS

- 1 medjool date, pitted
- 1 orange, peeled and seeded
- 1 banana
- 1 cup frozen blueberries
- 1 tablespoon ground chia seeds
- 1 cup spinach, romaine or any other greens

DIRECTIONS

Blend all ingredients together in a high powered blender until smooth and creamy.

PER SERVING: CALORIES 207; PROTEIN 2g; CARBOHYDRATES 49g; TOTAL FAT 2.4g; SATURATED FAT 0.3g; SODIUM 3mg; FIBER 8.7g; BETA-CAROTENE 131ug; VITAMIN C 77mg; CALCIUM 75mg; IRON 0.8mg; FOLATE 62ug; MAGNESIUM 52mg; ZINC 0.4mg; SELENIUM 2.6ug

CHOCOLATE SMOOTHIE

Serves: 2

INGREDIENTS

    5 ounces baby spinach

    2 cups frozen blueberries

    1/2 cup unsweetened soy, hemp or almond milk

    1 banana

    4 dates, pitted

    2 tablespoons natural cocoa powder

    1 tablespoon ground flax seeds

DIRECTIONS

Blend all ingredients in a high powered blender until smooth and creamy.

PER SERVING: CALORIES 276; PROTEIN 8g; CARBOHYDRATES 60g; TOTAL FAT 4.8g; SATURATED FAT 0.9g; SODIUM 93mg; FIBER 12.2g; BETA-CAROTENE 4288ug; VITAMIN C 29mg; CALCIUM 139mg; IRON 4.3mg; FOLATE 178ug; MAGNESIUM 147mg; ZINC 1.4mg; SELENIUM 5.9ug

CHOCOLATE CHERRY SMOOTHIE

Serves: 2

INGREDIENTS

4 ounces baby spinach

1/2 cup unsweetened soy, hemp or almond milk

1/2 cup pomegranate juice, cherry juice or cherry pomegranate juice

1 tablespoon natural cocoa powder

1 cup frozen cherries

1 banana

1 cup frozen blueberries

1/2 teaspoon vanilla extract

2 tablespoons ground flax seeds

DIRECTIONS

Blend all ingredients in a high powered blender until smooth and creamy.

PER SERVING: CALORIES 270; PROTEIN 8g; CARBOHYDRATES 53g; TOTAL FAT 5.5g; SATURATED FAT 0.8g; SODIUM 84mg; FIBER 9.9g; BETA-CAROTENE 3475ug; VITAMIN C 28mg; CALCIUM 119mg; IRON 3.5mg; FOLATE 147ug; MAGNESIUM 128mg; ZINC 1.2mg; SELENIUM 6.2ug

Eat Your Greens Fruit Smoothie

Serves: 2

INGREDIENTS

5 ounces baby spinach

1 banana

1 cup frozen or fresh blueberries

1/2 cup unsweetened soy, hemp or almond milk

1/2 cup pomegranate juice or other unsweetened fruit juice

1 tablespoon ground flaxseeds

DIRECTIONS

Blend all ingredients in a high powered blender until smooth and creamy.

PER SERVING: CALORIES 196; PROTEIN 6g; CARBOHYDRATES 39g; TOTAL FAT 3.6g; SATURATED FAT 0.4g; SODIUM 94mg; FIBER 6.9g; BETA-CAROTENE 4245ug; VITAMIN C 34mg; CALCIUM 111mg; IRON 3.3mg; FOLATE 167ug; MAGNESIUM 105mg; ZINC 0.9mg; SELENIUM 5.1ug

SUPER EASY BLENDED SALAD

Serves: 1

INGREDIENTS

- 8 ounces baby greens
- 1 orange, peeled and seeded
- 1 tablespoon fresh lemon juice

DIRECTIONS

Blend ingredients in a high powered blender until smooth and creamy.

PER SERVING: CALORIES 106; PROTEIN 4g; CARBOHYDRATES 24g; TOTAL FAT 0.8g; SATURATED FAT 0.1g;
SODIUM 39mg; FIBER 7g; BETA-CAROTENE 316ug; VITAMIN C 96mg; CALCIUM 168mg;
IRON 1.6mg; FOLATE 254ug; MAGNESIUM 54mg; ZINC 1.2mg; SELENIUM 0.7ug

TROPICAL MINT SMOOTHIE

Serves: 1

INGREDIENTS

1/2 cup fresh or frozen pineapple

1 cup fresh mango, peeled and cut into chunks or frozen mango

2 medium oranges, peeled and seeded

1 cup baby spinach

6 large mint leaves

DIRECTIONS

Blend all ingredients in a high powered blender until smooth and creamy.

PER SERVING: CALORIES 139; PROTEIN 2g; CARBOHYDRATES 35g; TOTAL FAT 0.5g; SATURATED FAT 0.1g; SODIUM 16mg; FIBER 5.6g; BETA-CAROTENE 1507ug; VITAMIN C 116mg; CALCIUM 86mg; IRON 1mg; FOLATE 91ug; MAGNESIUM 39mg; ZINC 0.3mg; SELENIUM 1.3ug

HIGH CRUCIFEROUS JUICE

Serves: 2

INGREDIENTS

- 3 medium carrots
- 3 cauliflower florets
- 1 apple, cored and cut in fourths
- 1/2 bunch kale
- 2/3 cup watercress
- 2 cups broccoli with stems

DIRECTIONS

Run all ingredients through a juicer.

PER SERVING: CALORIES 64; PROTEIN 3.5g; CARBOHYDRATES 14g; TOTAL FAT 0.4g; SATURATED FAT 0g;
SODIUM 61mg; FIBER 3.9g; BETA-CAROTENE 5828ug; VITAMIN C 73mg; CALCIUM 74mg;
IRON 0.8mg; FOLATE 50ug; MAGNESIUM 26mg; ZINC 0.4mg; SELENIUM 1.4ug

MIXED VEGETABLE JUICE

Serves: 2

INGREDIENTS

4 kale leaves

5 carrots, peeled

2 stalks bok choy

1 apple, cored and cut in quarters

1 medium beets, peeled

2/3 cup watercress with stems

DIRECTIONS

Run all ingredients through a juicer.

PER SERVING: CALORIES 80; PROTEIN 4g; CARBOHYDRATES 18g; TOTAL FAT 0.5g; SATURATED FAT 0g; SODIUM 93mg; FIBER 4.6g; BETA-CAROTENE 9581ug; VITAMIN C 55mg; CALCIUM 99mg; IRON 1.2mg; FOLATE 58ug; MAGNESIUM 32mg; ZINC 0.5mg; SELENIUM .75ug

Refreshing Sunrise Juice

Serves: 2

INGREDIENTS

2 cups fresh pineapple

1 cup baby carrots

1/8 slice lemon, without rind

1 tablespoon Goji berries

1 cup ice cubes

DIRECTIONS

Blend all ingredients together in a high-powered blender.

PER SERVING: CALORIES 110; PROTEIN 1g; CARBOHYDRATES 28g; TOTAL FAT 0.3g; SODIUM 49mg; FIBER 3.5g; BETA-CAROTENE 3887ug; VITAMIN C 63mg; CALCIUM 42mg; IRON 1.1mg; FOLATE 44ug; MAGNESIUM 26mg; ZINC 0.3mg; SELENIUM 0./ug

BREAKFAST

APPLE SUPREME

Serves: 4

INGREDIENTS

6 apples, cored, peeled, and chopped, divided

2 teaspoons cinnamon

1/2 cup chopped walnuts

3 dates, pitted

2 tablespoons ground flax seed

1/4 cup unsweetened soy, almond or hemp milk

1/2 cup raisins

1/2 cup old fashioned oats

DIRECTIONS

Preheat oven to 350° F.

In a high-powered blender, combine one cup of the chopped apples with cinnamon, walnuts, dates, flax seed and soy milk. Pour over remaining chopped apples. Add raisins and mix well. Sprinkle oats on top. Bake for 15 minutes.

PER SERVING: CALORIES 331; PROTEIN 10g; CARBOHYDRATES 58g; TOTAL FAT 11.8g; SATURATED FAT 1.2g; SODIUM 13mg; FIBER 9.1g; BETA-CAROTENE 113ug; VITAMIN C 10mg; CALCIUM 55mg; IRON 2mg; FOLATE 31ug; MAGNESIUM 80mg; ZINC 1.1mg; SELENIUM 5.6ug

ANTIOXIDANT-RICH BREAKFAST BARS

Serves: 6

INGREDIENTS

- 1 medium ripe banana
- 1 cup old fashioned oats
- 1 cup frozen blueberries, thawed
- 1/4 cup raisins
- 1/8 cup pomegranate juice
- 2 tablespoons finely chopped dates
- 1 tablespoon chopped walnuts
- 1 tablespoon Goji berries
- 1 tablespoon raw sunflower seeds
- 2 tablespoons ground flax seed

DIRECTIONS

Preheat oven to 350° F.

Mash banana in a large bowl. Add remaining ingredients and mix thoroughly.

Lightly wipe an 8 X 8 baking pan with a small amount of olive oil. Spread mixture into pan. Bake for 25 minutes. Cool on wire rack and cut into bars.

Refrigerate any leftover bars.

PER SERVING: CALORIES 146; PROTEIN 3g; CARBOHYDRATES 27g; TOTAL FAT 3.8g; SATURATED FAT 0.4g; SODIUM 2mg; FIBER 4g; BETA-CAROTENE 13ug; VITAMIN C 3mg; CALCIUM 17mg; IRON 1.2mg; FOLATE 19ug; MAGNESIUM 63mg; ZINC 0.7mg; SELENIUM 6.5ug

BANANA CASHEW LETTUCE WRAP

Serves: 2

INGREDIENTS

1/4 cup raw cashew butter

12 romaine lettuce leaves

2 bananas, thinly sliced

DIRECTIONS

Spread about 1 teaspoon cashew butter on each lettuce leaf. Lay a few banana slices on the butter and roll up like a burrito.

Note: This makes a delicious, healthy breakfast or snack.

PER SERVING: CALORIES 312; PROTEIN 8g; CARBOHYDRATES 39g; TOTAL FAT 16.5g; SATURATED FAT 3.3g; SODIUM 15mg; FIBER 6.1g; BETA-CAROTENE 3933ug; VITAMIN C 37mg; CALCIUM 57mg; IRON 3mg; FOLATE 198ug; MAGNESIUM 130mg; ZINC 2.1mg; SELENIUM 5.3ug

BERRY "YOGURT"

Serves: 2

INGREDIENTS

2 cups fresh or frozen blueberries, blackberries or strawberries

3/4 cup soy, almond or hemp milk

2 tablespoons ground flax or chia seeds

4 dates, pitted

DIRECTIONS

Add all ingredients to high powered blender and blend until smooth. Chill before serving.

May be served over fresh or thawed frozen berries.

PER SERVING: CALORIES 214; PROTEIN 25g; CARBOHYDRATES 42g; TOTAL FAT 5.2g; SATURATED FAT 0.5g; SODIUM 53mg; FIBER 7.9g; BETA-CAROTENE 378ug; VITAMIN C 14mg; CALCIUM 67mg; IRON 2mg; FOLATE 32ug; MAGNESIUM 66mg; ZINC 1mg; SELENIUM 6.7ug

CINNAMON FRUIT OATMEAL

Serves: 2

INGREDIENTS

1 cup water

1 teaspoon vanilla extract

1/4 teaspoon cinnamon

1/2 cup old-fashioned rolled oats

1/2 cup blueberries

2 apples, chopped

2 tablespoons chopped walnuts

1 tablespoon ground flax seeds

1/4 cup raisins

DIRECTIONS

In a saucepan, combine water with the vanilla and cinnamon. Bring to a boil over high heat. Reduce the heat to a simmer and stir in the oats.

When the mixture starts to simmer, add the blueberries. Remove from heat when berries are heated through.

Cover and let stand for 15 minutes until thick and creamy.

Mix in apples, nuts, flax seeds, and raisins.

PER SERVING: CALORIES 241; PROTEIN 13g; CARBOHYDRATES 41g; TOTAL FAT 8.1g; SATURATED FAT 0.8g; SODIUM 7mg; FIBER 7.8g; BETA-CAROTENE 50ug; VITAMIN C 10mg; CALCIUM 34mg; IRON 1.7mg; FOLATE 25ug; MAGNESIUM 90mg; ZINC 1.1mg; SELENIUM 8.1ug

DELUXE TOFU SCRAMBLE

Serves: 2

INGREDIENTS

3 whole scallions, diced

1/2 cup finely chopped red bell pepper

1 medium tomato, chopped

2 cloves garlic, minced or pressed

2 cups firm tofu, drained and crumbled

1 tablespoon Dr. Fuhrman's VegiZest
or other no salt seasoning blend, adjusted to taste

1/2 teaspoon Mrs. Dash no salt seasoning

1 tablespoon nutritional yeast

5 ounces baby spinach, coarsely chopped

1 teaspoon Bragg Liquid Aminos

DIRECTIONS

In a large skillet, over medium/high heat, sauté scallions, red pepper, tomato, and garlic in 1/4 cup water for 5 minutes.

Add remaining ingredients and cook for another 5 minutes.

PER SERVING: CALORIES 164; PROTEIN 12g; CARBOHYDRATES 28g; TOTAL FAT 2.7g; SATURATED FAT 0.3g; CHOLESTEROL 0.1mg; SODIUM 218mg; FIBER 5.1g; BETA-CAROTENE 5901ug; VITAMIN C 87mg; CALCIUM 202mg; IRON 5.3mg; FOLATE 355ug; MAGNESIUM 112mg; ZINC 1.7mg; SELENIUM 14.2ug

DR. FUHRMAN'S FRUIT, NUT, & VEGGIE BREAKFAST

Serves: 3

INGREDIENTS

1/4 cup diced fennel bulb

1 medium cucumber, peeled, thinly sliced in rounds & halved

1 cup blueberries

1 cup organic strawberries, sliced

1 green apple, peeled and sliced

1/4 cup chopped walnuts

For the Sauce:

1/2 cup raw cashews or 1/4 cup raw cashew butter

1/2 cup unsweetened soy, hemp or almond milk

3 dates, pitted

DIRECTIONS

Combine vegetables, fruits, and nuts.

Blend sauce ingredients in a high-powered blender until smooth.

Pour sauce over vegetable/fruit mixture and toss.

PER SERVING: CALORIES 318; PROTEIN 9g; CARBOHYDRATES 36g; TOTAL FAT 18.5g; SATURATED FAT 2.8g; SODIUM 33mg; FIBER 6.9g; BETA-CAROTENE 208ug; VITAMIN C 36mg; CALCIUM 69mg; IRON 2.8mg; FOLATE 65ug; MAGNESIUM 112mg; ZINC 2.1mg; SELENIUM 5.7ug

OATMEAL WITH FRUIT COMPOTE

Serves: 2

INGREDIENTS

3 cups fresh chopped assorted fruit

1/4 cup raisins or other dried fruit, chopped

orange juice or pomegranate juice

1 cup old fashioned rolled oats

1 cup soy, hemp or almond milk

DIRECTIONS

To make fruit compote: Combine the fresh and dried fruits in a glass jar along with enough juice to just cover the fruit. Cover and refrigerate overnight.

Combine oats and soy milk, cover and refrigerate overnight.

In the morning, top oats with fruit compote.

PER SERVING: CALORIES 322; PROTEIN 7g; CARBOHYDRATES 70g; TOTAL FAT 3.5g; SATURATED FAT 0.5g; SODIUM 43mg; FIBER 6.8g; BETA-CAROTENE 4848ug; VITAMIN C 95mg; CALCIUM 31mg IRON 2.9mg; FOLATE 67ug; MAGNESIUM 143mg; ZINC 1.8mg; SELENIUM 14.7ug

PHYTO-BLAST BREAKFAST BOWL

Serves: 2

INGREDIENTS

- 1 apple, cut into slices
- 1 banana, sliced
- 1 orange, sectioned
- 1/2 cup blueberries
- 1/2 cup sliced organic strawberries
- 2 tablespoons ground chia, hemp or flax seeds
- 2 tablespoons raw chopped walnuts

DIRECTIONS

Combine fruit and berries. Add seeds and nuts and toss.

PER SERVING: CALORIES 252; PROTEIN 6g; CARBOHYDRATES 42g; TOTAL FAT 10g; SATURATED FAT 0.9g; SODIUM 5mg; FIBER 7.8g; BETA-CAROTENE 96ug; VITAMIN C 68mg; CALCIUM 68mg; IRON 1.1mg; FOLATE 54ug; MAGNESIUM 69mg; ZINC 0.8mg; SELENIUM 1.7ug

POMEGRANATE MUESLI

Serves: 2

INGREDIENTS

- 1/2 cup pomegranate juice
- 1/4 cup steel cut or old fashioned oats (not quick or instant)
- 1 apple, peeled and grated
- 4 raw cashews or hazelnuts, coarsely chopped
- 1/2 cup halved grapes
- 1/2 cup cubed cantaloupe
- 1/2 cup sliced organic strawberries
- 1 tablespoon dried currants
- 1 tablespoon ground flax seeds

DIRECTIONS

Soak oats in pomegranate juice overnight in refrigerator. Oats will absorb the liquid.

In the morning, combine oats with remaining ingredients.

Note: You may add or substitute any fruits according to taste.

PER SERVING: CALORIES 258; PROTEIN 7g; CARBOHYDRATES 44g; TOTAL FAT 8.7g; SATURATED FAT 1.4g; SODIUM 13mg; FIBER 5.5g; BETA-CAROTENE 844ug; VITAMIN C 50mg; CALCIUM 31mg; IRON 2.3mg; FOLATE 30ug; MAGNESIUM 97mg; ZINC 1.5mg; SELENIUM 7.4ug

QUICK BANANA BERRY BREAKFAST TO GO

Serves: 2

INGREDIENTS

> 2 cups fresh or frozen blueberries
>
> 2 bananas, sliced
>
> 1/2 cup old-fashioned rolled oats
>
> 1/3 cup pomegranate juice
>
> 1-2 tablespoons chopped walnuts
>
> 1 tablespoon raw sunflower seeds
>
> 2 tablespoons dried currants

DIRECTIONS

Combine all ingredients in a small microwave-proof bowl. Heat in the microwave for 3 minutes.

Note: On the go, combine all ingredients in a sealed container and eat later, either hot or cold.

PER SERVING: CALORIES 362; PROTEIN 6g; CARBOHYDRATES 74g; TOTAL FAT 7.5g; SATURATED FAT 0.9g; SODIUM 5mg; FIBER 10.6g; BETA-CAROTENE 80ug; VITAMIN C 15mg; CALCIUM 35mg; IRON 2.2mg; FOLATE 57ug; MAGNESIUM 119mg; ZINC 1.3mg; SELENIUM 11.1ug

QUINOA BREAKFAST

Serves: 4

INGREDIENTS

1 cup quinoa, rinsed well*

2 cups water

1 cup unsweetened soy, hemp or almond milk

1/4 cup chopped prunes

1/4 cup frozen wild blueberries

1/4 cup chopped dried apricots, unsulphured

1/4 cup raisins

1/4 cup chopped dates

1/2 teaspoon ground cinnamon

1/4 teaspoon ground coriander

1/4 cup chopped Brazil nuts

DIRECTIONS

Simmer the quinoa in the water for 10 minutes. When water is absorbed completely, add the remaining ingredients and simmer another 10 minutes until soy milk is absorbed.

* *Be sure to rinse the quinoa well, using a small screen strainer, since some of the bitter coating may not have been removed during processing.*

PER SERVING: CALORIES 357; PROTEIN 10g; CARBOHYDRATES 62g; TOTAL FAT 9.7g; SATURATED FAT 1.7g; SODIUM 48mg; FIBER 6.9g; BETA-CAROTENE 441ug; VITAMIN C 1mg; CALCIUM 88mg; IRON 5.5mg; FOLATE 37ug; MAGNESIUM 154mg; ZINC 2.2mg; SELENIUM 171.2ug

SPECIAL OATMEAL

Serves: 4

INGREDIENTS

1 3/4 cups water

1 cup old-fashioned oats

4 dates, pitted and chopped

1/4 teaspoon coriander

2 bananas, sliced

1 cup chopped or grated apple

1 cup fresh or frozen blueberries

2 tablespoons ground flax seeds

DIRECTIONS

In a saucepan, bring the water to a boil and stir in all ingredients except blueberries and ground flax seeds. Simmer for 5 minutes.

Stir in blueberries. Sprinkle flax seeds on top or stir in. Cover for 2-3 minutes before serving.

If desired, this recipe may be made in the oven:

Preheat oven to 350° F. In a baking dish, combine water, oats, dates and coriander. Bake uncovered for 30 minutes. Add the bananas and more water, if desired. Bake another 15 minutes. Stir in apple and blueberries. Sprinkle flax seeds on top.

PER SERVING: CALORIES 280; PROTEIN 9g; CARBOHYDRATES 55g; TOTAL FAT 4.7g; SATURATED FAT 0.7g; SODIUM 6mg; FIBER 9g; BETA-CAROTENE 35ug; VITAMIN C 7mg; CALCIUM 44mg; IRON 2.4mg; FOLATE 42ug; MAGNESIUM 107mg; ZINC 1.9mg; SELENIUM 11.8ug

TROPICAL FRUIT SALAD

Serves: 4

INGREDIENTS

2 cups cubed pineapple

1 cup cubed mango

1 cup cubed papaya

2 oranges, peeled and sliced

1 banana, sliced

2 tablespoons unsweetened shredded coconut

shredded romaine lettuce

DIRECTIONS

Toss fruit together. Add coconut and serve on top of lettuce.

Serve immediately.

PER SERVING: CALORIES 146; PROTEIN 2g; CARBOHYDRATES 36g; TOTAL FAT 1.3g; SATURATED FAT 0.8g; SODIUM 5mg; FIBER 5.3g; BETA-CAROTENE 848ug; VITAMIN C 102mg; CALCIUM 55mg; IRON 0.6mg; FOLATE 76ug; MAGNESIUM 34mg; ZINC 0.3mg; SELENIUM 1.5ug

Wild Blueberry Hot Breakfast

Serves: 2

INGREDIENTS

2 cups frozen wild blueberries

1/2 cup unsweetened soy, hemp or almond milk

1/4 cup unsweetened shredded coconut, lightly toasted

1/4 cup chopped walnuts

1/4 cup dried currants

1 banana, sliced

DIRECTIONS

Heat frozen blueberries and soy milk until warm. Add remaining ingredients and stir well.

PER SERVING: CALORIES 345; PROTEIN 7g; CARBOHYDRATES 52g; TOTAL FAT 15.3g; SATURATED FAT 4.2g; SODIUM 39mg; FIBER 9.6g; BETA-CAROTENE 288ug; VITAMIN C 10mg; CALCIUM 69mg; IRON 2.3mg; FOLATE 51ug; MAGNESIUM 72mg; ZINC 1.1mg; SELENIUM 5.5ug

SALADS

APPLE BOK CHOY SALAD

Serves: 4

INGREDIENTS

6 cups finely chopped bok choy

1 large apple, shredded

1 large carrot, shredded

1/2 cup chopped red onion

1/2 cup unsweetened soy, hemp or almond milk

1/2 cup raw cashews or 1/4 cup raw cashew butter

1/4 cup balsamic vinegar

1/4 cup raisins

1 teaspoon Dijon mustard

DIRECTIONS

Combine bok choy, apple, carrot and chopped onion in a large bowl.

Blend soy milk, cashews, vinegar, raisins and mustard in a food processor or high powered blender. Add desired amount to chopped vegetables.

PER SERVING: CALORIES 202; PROTEIN 7g; CARBOHYDRATES 26g; TOTAL FAT 8.9g; SATURATED FAT 1.7g; SODIUM 89mg; FIBER 4g; BETA-CAROTENE 1383ug; VITAMIN C 20mg; CALCIUM 90mg; IRON 2.3mg; FOLATE 55ug; MAGNESIUM 74mg; ZINC 1.4mg; SELENIUM 4.2ug

BLACK BEAN MANGO SALAD

Serves: 6

INGREDIENTS

1 mango, peeled, pitted and cubed

2 tablespoons chopped fresh cilantro

4 green onions, thinly sliced

1 medium red bell pepper, seeded and chopped

1 cup frozen corn, thawed or fresh corn off the cob

3 cups cooked black beans* or 2 (15 ounce) cans black beans, no-salt-added or low sodium, drained

3 tablespoons fresh lime juice

1 teaspoon minced fresh garlic

1 teaspoon dried oregano

1 teaspoon ground cumin

dash chili powder

9 cups chopped romaine lettuce

DIRECTIONS

If using fresh corn on the cob, steam for 7 minutes or until tender, drain, cool and cut kernels off the cob, cutting close to the cob.

Mix all the ingredients, except the lettuce. Allow salad to stand at least 15 minutes before serving. Serve on a bed of chopped green lettuce.

The vegetable mixture can be made a day ahead and refrigerated. To do so, combine all the ingredients except the mango. Add the mango and a splash of lime juice just before serving.

* *Use 1 cup dried beans. See cooking instructions on page 195.*

PER SERVING: CALORIES 279; PROTEIN 16g; CARBOHYDRATES 55g; TOTAL FAT 1.7g; SATURATED FAT 0.3g; SODIUM 17mg; FIBER 17.7g; BETA-CAROTENE 5005ug; VITAMIN C 91mg; CALCIUM 106mg; IRON 4.9mg; FOLATE 398ug; MAGNESIUM 135mg; ZINC 2.2mg; SELENIUM 2.9ug

BROCCOLI AND SPINACH MICROSALAD

Serves: 2

INGREDIENTS

- 4 ounces spinach
- 1 pear, cored and quartered
- 1 Granny Smith apple, cored and quartered
- 1 lime, peeled
- 1/4 cup walnuts
- 4 cups broccoli florets

DIRECTIONS

Place spinach on the bottom of a 14 cup food processor. Add pear, apple and lime. Place broccoli, then nuts on top. Chop with the S blade until coarse but evenly chopped.

PER SERVING: CALORIES 265; PROTEIN 11g; CARBOHYDRATES 42g; TOTAL FAT 10.7g; SATURATED FAT 1g; SODIUM 107mg; FIBER 12.1g; BETA-CAROTENE 3888ug; VITAMIN C 195mg; CALCIUM 179mg; IRON 3.7mg; FOLATE 250ug; MAGNESIUM 117mg; ZINC 1.6mg; SELENIUM 6.1ug

CITRUS SALAD
WITH ORANGE PEANUT DRESSING

Serves: 4

INGREDIENTS

DRESSING

> 1/2 cup orange juice
>
> 1/4 cup unsalted lightly roasted peanuts or 1/8 cup unsalted natural peanut butter
>
> 1/4 cup raw cashews or 1/8 cup raw cashew butter
>
> 2 tablespoons rice vinegar
>
> 1 teaspoon Bragg Liquid Aminos or low sodium soy sauce
>
> 1/4 inch piece fresh ginger, peeled
>
> 1 clove garlic, chopped

SALAD

> 15 ounces or 10 cups baby lettuce mix
>
> 1 ripe avocado, peeled, pitted and sliced
>
> 1 orange, peeled and sliced
>
> 1/2 small sweet onion, cut in half and thinly sliced
>
> 1 tablespoon unhulled sesame seeds, lightly toasted*

DIRECTIONS

> Blend all dressing ingredients in high powered blender or food processor until smooth.
>
> To prepare salad, arrange avocado slices, onions, and orange rounds on top of lettuce.
>
> Pour dressing over salad and sprinkle with sesame seeds.

*Lightly toast sesame seeds in a pan over medium heat for two minutes, shaking pan frequently.

PER SERVING: CALORIES 409; PROTEIN 12g; CARBOHYDRATES 40g; TOTAL FAT 26.3g; SATURATED FAT 5.1g; SODIUM 92mg; FIBER 17.8g; BETA-CAROTENE 9894ug; VITAMIN C 146mg; CALCIUM 156mg; IRON 4.1mg; FOLATE 484ug; MAGNESIUM 136mg; ZINC 2.4mg; SELENIUM 3.2ug

DIJON VINAIGRETTE ASPARAGUS

Serves: 4

INGREDIENTS

2 pounds asparagus, tough ends removed

1/2 cup water

1/4 cup balsamic vinegar

1/4 cup walnuts

1/2 cup raisins

1 teaspoon Dijon mustard

2 cloves garlic, pressed

2 tablespoons chopped red onion

2 tablespoons pine nuts

DIRECTIONS

Place asparagus in a large skillet; add 1/2 inch of water. Bring to a boil, reduce heat; cover and simmer for 3-5 minutes until crisp-tender.

Drain asparagus and arrange in a shallow dish. Combine water, vinegar, walnuts, raisins, mustard and garlic in a food processor or high powered blender, stir in red onion and pour over asparagus. Let stand at room temperature for 1-2 hours before serving.

Sprinkle with pine nuts before serving.

PER SERVING: CALORIES 207; PROTEIN 7g; CARBOHYDRATES 28g; TOTAL FAT 8.1g; SATURATED FAT 0.8g; SODIUM 42mg; FIBER 6.2g; BETA-CAROTENE 1020ug; VITAMIN C 14mg; CALCIUM 80mg; IRON 5.8mg; FOLATE 128ug; MAGNESIUM 63mg; ZINC 1.8mg; SELENIUM 5.9ug

GREEK CHICKPEA SALAD

Serves: 4

INGREDIENTS

1 1/2 cups cooked garbanzo beans (chick peas)* or 1 (15 ounce) can garbanzo beans, no-salt-added or low sodium, drained

3 plum tomatoes, chopped

1 boiled potato, peeled and chopped in chunks

1 green apple, peeled, cored and chopped

1 cucumber, chopped

1/2 small onion, chopped

1/4 cup chopped Brazil nuts, divided

3 tablespoons Dr. Fuhrman's Spicy Pecan Vinegar or balsamic vinegar

1 tablespoon chopped cilantro

10 ounces mixed salad greens

DIRECTIONS

Mix all ingredients, except salad greens and 2 tablespoons Brazil nuts. Serve on bed of mixed salad greens and sprinkle with remaining Brazil nuts.

* Use 1/2 cup dry chick peas. See cooking instructions on page 195.

Note: This is even better when refrigerated overnight to blend flavors.

PER SERVING: CALORIES 288; PROTEIN 15g; CARBOHYDRATES 54g; TOTAL FAT 3.5g; SATURATED FAT 0.4g; SODIUM 23mg; FIBER 12.9g; BETA-CAROTENE 2821ug; VITAMIN C 36mg; CALCIUM 106mg; IRON 4.6mg; FOLATE 313ug; MAGNESIUM 94mg; ZINC 2.3mg; SELENIUM 4.9ug

GREENS AND BERRIES SALAD WITH CASHEW CURRANT DRESSING

Serves: 2

INGREDIENTS

CASHEW DRESSING

> 1/4 cup raw cashews or 2 tablespoons raw cashew butter
>
> 1/3 cup unsweetened soy, hemp or almond milk
>
> 1 apple, peeled and sliced
>
> 2 tablespoons dried currants or raisins

SALAD

> 1 head (about 6 cups) romaine lettuce
>
> 5 ounces (about 5 cups) baby spinach
>
> 1 (12-ounce) bag frozen strawberries, defrosted and sliced in half

DIRECTIONS

> To make dressing, blend cashews or cashew butter with soy milk and apple in a high powered blender until smooth. Add the currants and blend well.
>
> Pile the lettuce and spinach leaves on a plate and lay the strawberries on top. Pour the juice from the strawberries over the greens.
>
> Drizzle dressing over the greens and berries.

PER SERVING: CALORIES 285; PROTEIN 11g; CARBOHYDRATES 47g; TOTAL FAT 9.8g; SATURATED FAT 1.8g; SODIUM 99mg; FIBER 12g; BETA-CAROTENE 10056ug; VITAMIN C 134mg; CALCIUM 188mg; IRON 6.7mg; FOLATE 416ug; MAGNESIUM 160mg; ZINC 2.2mg; SELENIUM 6.6ug

SUPER SLAW

Serves: 3

INGREDIENTS

SLAW

> 2 cups shredded apples
>
> 1 cup shredded raw cabbage
>
> 1 cup shredded raw beets
>
> 1 cup shredded raw carrots
>
> 1/2 cup raisins

DRESSING

> 1/2 cup soft tofu
>
> 1/4 cup unsweetened soy, almond or hemp milk
>
> 1 tablespoon Dr. Fuhrman's Riesling Reserve Vinegar
>
> 1 tablespoon Dr. Fuhrman's Spicy Pecan Vinegar
>
> 3 dates, pitted
>
> 2 teaspoons fresh lemon juice
>
> 1/4 cup chopped pecans, lightly toasted *

DIRECTIONS

> Combine slaw ingredients.
>
> Blend dressing ingredients and toss with slaw. Top with toasted pecans.

* Lightly toast pecans in a 300 degree oven for 3 minutes.

PER SERVING: CALORIES 277; PROTEIN 6g; CARBOHYDRATES 52g; TOTAL FAT 7.7g; SATURATED FAT 0.7g; SODIUM 83mg; FIBER 7.3g; BETA-CAROTENE 3153ug; VITAMIN C 19mg; CALCIUM 80mg; IRON 2mg; FOLATE 82ug; MAGNESIUM 56mg; ZINC 1mg; SELENIUM 4.3ug

QUINOA BEAN SALAD

Serves: 6

INGREDIENTS

2 cups cooked quinoa

1 1/2 cups cooked white beans* or 1 (15 ounce) can white beans, no-salt-added or low sodium, drained

1 cup grated carrots

1 cup dried currants

1/2 cup walnuts, chopped

2 plum tomatoes, chopped

1 small red onion, thinly sliced

1/2 green bell pepper, chopped

1/2 red bell pepper, chopped

1/2 orange or yellow bell pepper, chopped

3 cloves garlic, minced

1 tablespoon chili powder

2 teaspoons Bragg Liquid Aminos or low sodium soy sauce

DIRECTIONS

Cook quinoa according to package directions.

Place all other ingredients in a large bowl and mix.

Add cooked quinoa and toss.

* *Use 1/2 cup dried beans. See cooking instructions on page 195.*

PER SERVING: CALORIES 383; PROTEIN 15g; CARBOHYDRATES 67g; TOTAL FAT 9g; SATURATED FAT 1g; CHOLESTEROL 0.1mg; SODIUM 122mg; FIBER 13.6g; BETA-CAROTENE 2018ug; VITAMIN C 58mg; CALCIUM 128mg; IRON 6.3mg; FOLATE 153ug; MAGNESIUM 149mg; ZINC 2.4mg; SELENIUM 2.2ug

SOUTHERN-STYLE MIXED GREENS SALAD

Serves: 2

INGREDIENTS

1 cup water

2 cloves garlic, minced

dash black pepper

1 1/2 cup cooked black eyed peas or other white bean*
or 1 (15 ounce) can no-salt added or low-sodium, drained

1 cup seeded and chopped yellow bell pepper

1 cup chopped fresh tomato

1/3 cup chopped fresh parsley

1/4 cup chopped red onion

2 tablespoons Dr. Fuhrman's Black Fig Vinegar or balsamic vinegar

10 ounces (about 7 cups) mixed salad greens

DIRECTIONS

Combine the water, garlic, and black pepper in a large saucepan; bring to a boil. Add black eyed peas; cover and simmer over low heat for 10 minutes. Drain.

In a bowl, combine the black eyed peas, bell pepper, tomato, parsley, onion, and vinegar. Cover and chill for 3 hours or overnight. Serve over the salad greens.

* Use 1/2 cup dry beans. See cooking instructions on page 195.

PER SERVING: CALORIES 390; PROTEIN 25g; CARBOHYDRATES 74g; TOTAL FAT 2.1g; SATURATED FAT 0.4g; SODIUM 39mg; FIBER 23.5g; BETA-CAROTENE 527ug; VITAMIN C 194mg; CALCIUM 201mg; IRON 6.2mg; FOLATE 536ug; MAGNESIUM 155mg; ZINC 3.1mg; SELENIUM 13.8ug

Spinach and Garbanzo Bean Salad with Lemon Fig Dressing

Serves: 4

INGREDIENTS

SALAD:

12 ounces baby spinach

1 1/2 cups cooked garbanzo beans* or 1 (15 ounce) can garbanzo beans, no-salt-added or low sodium, drained

1 cup shredded carrots

1 cup broccoli florets

1 cup mushrooms, thinly sliced

1 cup chopped tomatoes

DRESSING:

2 tablespoons fresh lemon juice

2 cloves garlic, minced

1/2 teaspoon dried parsley

1/2 teaspoon dried basil

1/4 teaspoon onion powder

1/4 teaspoon ground mustard seed

1/4 cup Dr. Fuhrman's Black Fig Vinegar or balsamic vinegar

DIRECTIONS

Whisk all dressing ingredients together. Pour over salad.

* Use 1/2 cup dry beans. See cooking instructions on page 195.

PER SERVING: CALORIES 237; PROTEIN 14g; CARBOHYDRATES 41g; TOTAL FAT 3.3g; SATURATED FAT 0.4g; SODIUM 46mg; FIBER 10.9g; BETA-CAROTENE 3648ug; VITAMIN C 135mg; CALCIUM 223mg; IRON 4.6mg; FOLATE 382ug; MAGNESIUM 138mg; ZINC 2.8mg; SELENIUM 14.2ug

TRIPLE TREAT CABBAGE SALAD

Serves: 4

INGREDIENTS

SALAD:

2 cups shredded green cabbage

1 cup shredded red cabbage

1 cup shredded savoy cabbage

1 carrot, peeled and grated

1 red pepper, thinly sliced

1/4 cup dried currants

2 tablespoons raw pumpkin seeds

2 tablespoons raw sunflower seeds

1 tablespoon unhulled sesame seeds

DRESSING:

1/3 cup unsweetened soy, almond or hemp milk

1 apple, peeled and sliced

1/2 cup raw cashews or 1/4 cup raw cashew butter

1 tablespoon Dr. Fuhrman's Spicy Pecan Vinegar or balsamic vinegar

1 tablespoon dried currants

1 tablespoon unhulled sesame seeds, lightly toasted*

DIRECTIONS

Mix all salad ingredients together.
In a high powered blender, blend soy milk, apple, cashews and vinegar and toss with salad.

Garnish with currants and lightly toasted sesame seeds.

* Lightly toast sesame seeds in a pan over medium heat for 2 minutes, shaking the pan frequently.

PER SERVING: CALORIES 239; PROTEIN 10g; CARBOHYDRATES 21g; TOTAL FAT 15g; SATURATED FAT 2.6g; SODIUM 49mg; FIBER 4.8g; BETA-CAROTENE 1636ug; VITAMIN C 33mg; CALCIUM 93mg; IRON 3.6mg; FOLATE 72ug; MAGNESIUM 129mg; ZINC 2.2mg; SELENIUM 7ug

WALNUT PEAR GREEN SALAD

Serves: 2

INGREDIENTS

8 ounces (about 5 cups) mixed baby greens

2 ounces (about 2 cups) arugula or watercress

1 pear, peeled, cored and grated

1/4 cup dried currants

1/4 cup chopped walnuts

2 tablespoons Dr. Fuhrman's D'Anjou Pear vinegar or rice vinegar

2 teaspoons olive oil

2 pears, peeled cored and sliced

1/4 cup walnut halves

DIRECTIONS

Combine the baby greens, arugula, grated pear, currants, and walnuts in a bowl. Toss with vinegar & olive oil. Top with sliced pears and walnut halves.

PER SERVING: CALORIES 367; PROTEIN 6g; CARBOHYDRATES 61g; TOTAL FAT 14.8g; SATURATED FAT 1.6g; SODIUM 29mg; FIBER 12.4g; BETA-CAROTENE 4792ug; VITAMIN C 51mg; CALCIUM 128mg; IRON 2.7mg; FOLATE 190ug; MAGNESIUM 72mg; ZINC 1.1mg; SELENIUM 1.8ug

DRESSINGS, DIPS, AND SAUCES

—DRESSINGS—

ALMOND BALSAMIC VINAIGRETTE

Serves: 6

INGREDIENTS

1/2 cup water

1/3 cup balsamic vinegar

1/4 cup raw almonds or 1/8 cup raw almond butter

1/4 cup raisins

6 cloves garlic, lightly roasted *(see note)*

1 teaspoon dried oregano

1/2 teaspoon dried basil

1/2 teaspoon onion powder

DIRECTIONS

Blend all ingredients in a food processor or high powered blender.

Note: Preheat oven to 350° F. Roast unpeeled garlic in a small baking dish for about 25 minutes or until soft.

PER SERVING: CALORIES 77; PROTEIN 2g; CARBOHYDRATES 10g; TOTAL FAT 3.1g; SATURATED FAT 0.2g; SODIUM 6mg; FIBER 1g; BETA-CAROTENE 13ug; VITAMIN C 1mg; CALCIUM 26mg; IRON 0.6mg; FOLATE 3ug; MAGNESIUM 22mg; ZINC 0.2mg; SELENIUM 0.5ug

BANANA WALNUT DRESSING/DIP

Serves: 2

INGREDIENTS

2 bananas

2 tablespoons walnuts

2 tablespoons raisins

1/4 cup Dr. Fuhrman's Riesling Reserve Vinegar or other fruit flavored vinegar

DIRECTIONS

Blend all ingredients in a high powered blender or food processor until smooth and creamy.

PER SERVING: CALORIES 104; PROTEIN 2g; CARBOHYDRATES 20g; TOTAL FAT 206g; SATURATED FAT 0.3g; SODIUM 5mg; FIBER 2g; BETA-CAROTENE 16ug; VITAMIN C 6mg; CALCIUM 13mg; IRON 0.5mg; FOLATE 15ug; MAGNESIUM 25mg; ZINC 0.2mg; SELENIUM 1.3ug

BLUEBERRY POMEGRANATE DRESSING

Serves: 4

INGREDIENTS

2 cups fresh or thawed frozen blueberries

1/2 cup pomegranate Juice

1/4 cup raw cashews

1/4 cup raw sunflower seeds

4 tablespoons Dr. Fuhrman's Blueberry Vinegar or other fruit-flavored vinegar

DIRECTIONS

Blend all ingredients in a high powered blender until smooth and creamy.

PER SERVING: CALORIES 162; PROTEIN 4g; CARBOHYDRATES 19g; TOTAL FAT 8.9g; SATURATED FAT 1.3g; SODIUM 5mg; FIBER 3.3g; BETA-CAROTENE 24ug; VITAMIN C 6mg; CALCIUM 21mg; IRON 1.5mg; FOLATE 32ug; MAGNESIUM 59mg; ZINC 1mg; SELENIUM 6.4ug

CASHEW CAESAR SALAD DRESSING

Serves: 4

INGREDIENTS

6 cloves garlic, roasted

2/3 cup unsweetened soy, almond or hemp milk

2/3 cup raw cashews or 1/3 cup raw cashew butter

1 1/2 tablespoons nutritional yeast

1 tablespoon plus 1 teaspoon fresh lemon juice

2 teaspoons Dijon mustard

black pepper, to taste

DIRECTIONS

Preheat the oven to 350° F. Break the garlic cloves apart, leaving on the papery skins. Roast for about 25 minutes or until soft.

When cool, remove the skins and blend with the remaining ingredients in a food processor or high powered blender until creamy and smooth.

Note: May be used for a veggie dip or pour over 2 chopped heads (12 cups) of romaine for a Caesar Salad for two.

PER SERVING: CALORIES 183; PROTEIN 10g; CARBOHYDRATES 11g; TOTAL FAT 11.4g; SATURATED FAT 2.2g; SODIUM 536mg; FIBER 1.3g; BETA-CAROTENE 147ug; VITAMIN C 3mg; CALCIUM 31mg; IRON 1.9mg; FOLATE 248ug; MAGNESIUM 70mg; ZINC 1.5mg; SELENIUM 5ug

DIJON PISTACHIO DRESSING/DIP

Serves: 4

INGREDIENTS

1 1/3 cups water

1 cup raw pistachio nuts

4 tablespoons lemon juice

2 tablespoons ground flax seeds

4 teaspoons Dr. Fuhrman's VegiZest
or other no salt seasoning blend, adjusted to taste

2 teaspoons Dijon mustard

1 teaspoon Bragg Liquid Aminos

1/2 teaspoon garlic powder

4 dates, pitted

DIRECTIONS

Blend all ingredients in a high powered blender or food processor until smooth and creamy. Add water as needed to achieve desired consistency.

PER SERVING: CALORIES 237; PROTEIN 8g; CARBOHYDRATES 21g; TOTAL FAT 15.2g; SATURATED FAT 1.8g; SODIUM 138mg; FIBER 5g; BETA-CAROTENE 513ug; VITAMIN C 10mg; CALCIUM 53mg; IRON 1.8mg; FOLATE 23ug; MAGNESIUM 59mg; ZINC 0.9mg; SELENIUM 3.1ug

GINGER ALMOND DRESSING

Serves: 3

INGREDIENTS

1/2 cup raw almonds or 1/4 cup raw almond butter

1/4 cup unsweetened soy, hemp or almond milk

1/4 cup water

2 tablespoons tahini or unhulled sesame seeds

3 dates, pitted

2 small cloves garlic, chopped

1/2 inch piece fresh ginger, peeled and chopped

DIRECTIONS

Blend all ingredients together in a high powered blender until creamy. Add more water if a thinner dressing is desired.

PER SERVING: CALORIES 238; PROTEIN 8g; CARBOHYDRATES 15g; TOTAL FAT 18g; SATURATED FAT 1.7g; SODIUM 23mg; FIBER 4g; BETA-CAROTENE 75ug; VITAMIN C 1mg; CALCIUM 82mg; IRON 1.7mg; FOLATE 22ug; MAGNESIUM 86mg; ZINC 1.4mg; SELENIUM 2.4ug

ORANGE SESAME DRESSING

Serves: 2

INGREDIENTS

1/4 cup unhulled sesame seeds, divided

1/4 cup raw cashew nuts or 1/8 cup raw cashew butter

1/2 cup orange juice

2 tablespoons Dr. Fuhrman's Riesling Reserve Vinegar or balsamic vinegar

2 oranges, peeled and diced

DIRECTIONS

Toast the sesame seeds in a dry skillet over medium high heat for 2 minutes, shaking the pan frequently. In a high powered blender, combine 2 tablespoons of the sesame seeds, cashews, orange juice, and vinegar.

Toss salad with dressing and diced oranges. Sprinkle the remaining sesame seeds on top.

Note: This tastes great on a spinach and mushroom salad with thinly sliced red onions.

PER SERVING: CALORIES 194; PROTEIN 5g; CARBOHYDRATES 18g; TOTAL FAT 12.5g; SATURATED FAT 2.2g; SODIUM 4mg; FIBER 3g; BETA-CAROTENE 57ug; VITAMIN C 50mg; CALCIUM 124mg; IRON 2.3mg; FOLATE 49ug; MAGNESIUM 83mg; ZINC 1.6mg; SELENIUM 2.7ug

RUSSIAN FIG DRESSING/DIP

Serves: 2

INGREDIENTS

1/3 cup no-salt-added or low sodium pasta sauce

1/3 cup raw almonds or 3 tablespoons raw almond butter

2 tablespoons raw sunflower seeds

3 tablespoons Dr. Fuhrman's Black Fig Vinegar

DIRECTIONS

Blend all ingredients in a food processor or high powered blender until smooth.

PER SERVING: CALORIES 227; PROTEIN 8g; CARBOHYDRATES 13g; TOTAL FAT 16.8g; SATURATED FAT 1.4g; SODIUM 17mg; FIBER 4g; BETA-CAROTENE 83ug; VITAMIN C 5mg; CALCIUM 74mg; IRON 2mg; FOLATE 31ug; MAGNESIUM 108mg; ZINC 1.3mg; SELENIUM 6.3ug

TEN THOUSAND ISLAND DRESSING

Serves: 4

INGREDIENTS

1 cup raw cashews or 1/2 cup raw cashew butter

1/2 cup unsweetened soy, almond or hemp milk

2 tablespoons balsamic vinegar

2 tablespoons lemon juice

1 teaspoon dried dill

1 teaspoon onion powder

1/2 teaspoon garlic powder

3 tablespoons tomato paste

2 dates, pitted

1 cucumber

1/4 cup finely chopped onion

DIRECTIONS

In food processor or high powered blender, blend the cashews, milk, vinegar, lemon juice, dill, onion powder, garlic powder, tomato paste, dates and cucumber until smooth. Transfer to a small bowl and fold in the finely chopped onion.

PER SERVING: CALORIES 254; PROTEIN 9g; CARBOHYDRATES 23g; TOTAL FAT 16.3g; SATURATED FAT 2.9g; SODIUM 120mg; FIBER 3g; BETA-CAROTENE 237ug; VITAMIN C 9mg; CALCIUM 47mg; IRON 3.4mg; FOLATE 25ug; MAGNESIUM 127mg; ZINC 2.4mg; SELENIUM 9.4ug

TOFU RANCH DRESSING/DIP

Serves: 4

INGREDIENTS

6 ounces silken tofu

3 dates, pitted

1 clove garlic, peeled

1/4 cup finely chopped green onion

3 tablespoons water

2 tablespoons lemon juice

1 1/2 tablespoons dried Italian seasoning

1 tablespoon chopped fresh parsley

1 tablespoon chopped fresh dill

1 teaspoon Bragg Liquid Aminos or low sodium soy sauce

dash cayenne pepper

DIRECTIONS

Blend all the ingredients in a high powered blender or food processor until smooth and creamy.

Note: Use as a dressing, dip, spread or mayonnaise substitute in your favorite recipes.

PER SERVING: CALORIES 63; PROTEIN 2g; CARBOHYDRATES 13g; TOTAL FAT 1g; SATURATED FAT 0.1g; CHOLESTEROL 0.1mg; SODIUM 65mg; FIBER 1.5g; BETA-CAROTENE 167ug; VITAMIN C 7mg; CALCIUM 72mg; IRON 1.5mg; FOLATE 24ug; MAGNESIUM 21mg; ZINC 0.4mg; SELENIUM 5ug

ZESTY AVOCADO DRESSING/DIP

Serves: 4

INGREDIENTS

1 large tomato, sliced

1 ripe avocado, peeled and pitted

1/3 cup red onion, sliced

1/2 cup green pepper, sliced

2 cloves garlic

2 tablespoons fresh lemon juice

2 tablespoons Dr. Fuhrman's Riesling Reserve Vinegar or balsamic vinegar

1 tablespoon Dr. Fuhrman's VegiZest or other no salt seasoning blend, adjusted to taste

DIRECTIONS

Blend all ingredients in a high powered blender or food processor until smooth. Add water if needed to achieve desired consistency.

PER SERVING: CALORIES 121; PROTEIN 4g; CARBOHYDRATES 13g; TOTAL FAT 7.8g; SATURATED FAT 1.5g; SODIUM 15mg; FIBER 5.3g; BETA-CAROTENE 781ug; VITAMIN C 47mg; CALCIUM 18mg; IRON 0.5mg; FOLATE 43ug; MAGNESIUM 26mg; ZINC 0.4mg; SELENIUM 0.3ug

BAKED GARLIC PITA CHIPS

Serves: 4

INGREDIENTS

2 (100% whole grain) pitas

olive oil cooking spray

garlic powder

DIRECTIONS

Preheat oven to 375° F.

Split each pita in half horizontally. Spray pita halves lightly with olive oil, if desired, and sprinkle with garlic powder.

Cut each half in half and then into four sections to form triangles.

Place on baking sheet and bake for 8 minutes or until lightly browned and crispy.

Serve with salsa or hummus.

PER SERVING: CALORIES 85; PROTEIN 3g; CARBOHYDRATES 18g; TOTAL FAT 0.8g; SATURATED FAT 0.1g; SODIUM 170mg; FIBER 2.4g; CALCIUM 5mg; IRON 1mg; FOLATE 11ug; MAGNESIUM 22mg; ZINC 0.5mg; SELENIUM 14.1ug

BLACK BEAN HUMMUS

Serves: 6

INGREDIENTS

11/2 cup cooked black beans* or 1 (15 ounce) can black beans, no-salt-added or low sodium, drained

2 tablespoons water

2 tablespoons fresh lemon juice

2 tablespoons Dr. Fuhrman's VegiZest or other no salt seasoning blend, adjusted to taste

2 tablespoons raw tahini

2 teaspoons Bragg Liquid Aminos or low sodium soy sauce

1/2 teaspoon ground cumin

1/2 clove garlic, chopped

dash cayenne pepper or more to taste

dash paprika, for garnish

DIRECTIONS

Blend all ingredients, except the paprika, in food processor or high powered blender until smooth, scraping down the sides as needed. Add more seasoning to taste. Add more water to achieve desired consistency.

Garnish with paprika.

Note: Serve with raw vegetables like baby carrots, steamed asparagus spears, broccoli florets, zucchini, cucumber, and romaine lettuce leaves.

Use 1/2 cup dry beans. See cooking instructions on page 195.

PER SERVING: CALORIES 132; PROTEIN 7g; CARBOHYDRATES 18g; TOTAL FAT 4g; SATURATED FAT 0.6g; SODIUM 106mg; FIBER 6.4g; VITAMIN C 4mg; CALCIUM 51mg; IRON 1.6mg; FOLATE 105ug; MAGNESIUM 54mg; ZINC 1.1mg; SELENIUM 0.9ug

Fresh Beet Hummus

Serves: 4

INGREDIENTS

4 medium beets

1 cup cooked chick peas

1/4 cup unhulled sesame seeds

2 tablespoons water

2 tablespoons lemon juice

1 garlic clove

2 teaspoons ground cumin

pinch black pepper

DIRECTIONS

Scrub beets, cover with water in a sauce pan and simmer until tender, about 30 minutes. Peel when cool enough to handle.

Place beets, chick peas, sesame seeds, water, lemon juice, garlic, cumin and black pepper in a food processor or high powered blender and pulse until smooth.

Note: Serve on top of sliced cucumber or zucchini rounds or as a dip with assorted raw vegetables.

PER SERVING: CALORIES 162; PROTEIN 7g; CARBOHYDRATES 22g; TOTAL FAT 5.9g; SATURATED FAT 0.8g; SODIUM 71mg; FIBER 5.7g; BETA-CAROTENE 24ug; VITAMIN C 8mg; CALCIUM 133mg; IRON 3.2mg; FOLATE 170ug; MAGNESIUM 71mg; ZINC 1.6mg; SELENIUM 2.7ug

FRESH TOMATO SALSA

Serves: 8

INGREDIENTS

2 fresh tomatoes

1 small red onion

2 scallions

1 clove garlic

1/2 jalapeno pepper, seeded and minced

3 tablespoons chopped cilantro

3 tablespoons fresh lime or lemon juice

DIRECTIONS

Chop the tomatoes and red onion into equal-sized pieces. Finely chop the scallions, including green portions.

In a mixing bowl, stir together all ingredients.

Serve immediately or refrigerate in a tightly covered container for up to 3 days.

Yields: 2 cups

PER SERVING: CALORIES 15; PROTEIN 1g; CARBOHYDRATES 4g; TOTAL FAT 0.1g; SODIUM 4mg; FIBER 0.8g; BETA-CAROTENE 228ug; VITAMIN C 8mg; CALCIUM 12mg; IRON 0.2mg; FOLATE 12ug; MAGNESIUM 7mg; ZINC 0.1mg; SELENIUM 0.2ug

GRANDMA TILLIE'S EGGPLANT DIP

Serves: 4

INGREDIENTS

1 medium eggplant

1 large tomato, diced

1 green or red bell pepper, diced

1 large onion, diced

1 teaspoon Mrs. Dash or other no salt seasoning

1/4 cup dried currants

DIRECTIONS

Pierce the eggplant with a fork to prevent it from bursting while cooking. Roast in a 350° F oven for 45-60 minutes, turning once during the cooking time, until eggplant is very tender when poked with a fork.* Cooking time will vary depending on the size of the eggplant.

Heat 1/8 cup water in a skillet and water sauté tomato, pepper and onion until soft. Scoop out or peel the eggplant and blend it with the tomato mixture and seasoning. Stir in currents.

Note: Serve as a dip for raw vegetables or a topping for steamed vegetables

---

* *To roast eggplant in the microwave, cut in half vertically, put on a plate and cover with plastic wrap. Microwave on high for 5 minutes; reduce power to 30% and microwave for an additional 5 minutes.*

PER SERVING: CALORIES 83; PROTEIN 3g; CARBOHYDRATES 20g; TOTAL FAT 0.5g; SATURATED FAT 0.1g; SODIUM 7mg; FIBER 6.7g; BETA-CAROTENE 647ug; VITAMIN C 47mg; CALCIUM 32mg; IRON 0.9mg; FOLATE 55ug; MAGNESIUM 33mg; ZINC 0.5mg; SELENIUM 0.6ug

HERBED WHITE BEAN HUMMUS

Serves: 2

INGREDIENTS

2 cups cooked white beans* or canned white beans, no-salt added or low-sodium, drained

1 tablespoon fresh lemon Juice

2 tablespoons unhulled sesame seeds

2 tablespoons red wine vinegar

1/2 teaspoon Dijon mustard

2 tablespoons water

1/4 cup chopped fresh basil

2 tablespoons chopped fresh thyme

DIRECTIONS

Blend the beans, lemon juice, sesame seeds, vinegar, mustard, and water in a high-powered blender or food processor until smooth. Add the basil and thyme and pulse very briefly. Do not over-process; the herbs should be visible in small pieces.

* *Use 2/3 cup dry beans. See cooking instructions on page 195*

PER SERVING: CALORIES 180; PROTEIN 10g; CARBOHYDRATES 30g; TOTAL FAT 2.7g; SATURATED FAT 0.4g; SODIUM 23mg; FIBER 7.1g; BETA-CAROTENE 118ug; VITAMIN C 4mg; CALCIUM 149mg; IRON 4.9mg; FOLATE 92ug; MAGNESIUM 87mg; ZINC 1.9mg; SELENIUM 2.4ug

SESAME GINGER SAUCE

Serves: 4

INGREDIENTS

- 2/3 cup water
- 1/2 cup raw tahini
- 2 tablespoons fresh lemon juice
- 1 teaspoon white miso
- 1 tablespoon finely grated fresh ginger
- 2 dates, pitted
- 1 clove garlic, pressed
- pinch hot pepper flakes

DIRECTIONS

Blend all the ingredients in a food processor or a high powered blender. Add more water if needed to achieve the desired consistency.

Note: Serve with steamed or water sauteed vegetables. This sauce goes well with bok choy, asparagus or kale.

PER SERVING: CALORIES 189; PROTEIN 6g; CARBOHYDRATES 13g; TOTAL FAT 14.4g; SATURATED FAT 2g; SODIUM 69mg; FIBER 3.3g; VITAMIN C 4mg; CALCIUM 131mg; IRON 0.9mg; FOLATE 31ug; MAGNESIUM 32mg; ZINC 1.4mg; SELENIUM 0.2ug

SIMPLE GUACAMOLE

Serves: 4

INGREDIENTS

2 ripe avocados, peeled and pitted

1/2 cup finely chopped onion

1/4 cup minced fresh cilantro

2 tablespoons fresh lime juice

1/4 teaspoon ground cumin

1/4 teaspoon freshly ground black pepper

DIRECTIONS

Using a fork, mash the avocados in a small bowl. Add the remaining ingredients and stir well. Cover and chill.

PER SERVING: CALORIES 194; PROTEIN 4g; CARBOHYDRATES 15g; TOTAL FAT 15.4g; SATURATED FAT 3g; SODIUM 7mg; FIBER 9.1g; BETA-CAROTENE 248ug; VITAMIN C 32mg; CALCIUM 26mg; IRON 0.4mg; FOLATE 61ug; MAGNESIUM 41mg; ZINC 0.6mg; SELENIUM 0.2ug

SPICY BEAN SPREAD

Serves: 4

INGREDIENTS

1 1/2 cups cooked pinto beans* or 1 (15 ounce) can pinto beans, no-salt-added or low sodium, drained

1 teaspoon Dr. Fuhrman's Black Fig Vinegar or balsamic vinegar

1/4 cup water

1/2 teaspoon crushed red chili pepper

2 garlic cloves

1 pinch turmeric

DIRECTIONS

In a blender or food processor, puree ingredients until smooth and creamy.

Note: Serve with raw or lightly steamed vegetables or toasted pita bread with shredded raw greens.

* Use 1/2 cup dry beans. See cooking instructions on page 195.

PER SERVING: CALORIES 154; PROTEIN 10g; CARBOHYDRATES 28g; TOTAL FAT 0.7g; SATURATED FAT 0.1g; SODIUM 1mg; FIBER 9.6g; VITAMIN C 1mg; CALCIUM 50mg; IRON 2.3mg; FOLATE 183ug; MAGNESIUM 54mg; ZINC 1mg; SELENIUM 6.7ug

TASTY HUMMUS

Serves: 4

INGREDIENTS

1 cup cooked garbanzo beans* or canned garbanzo beans, no-salt-added or low sodium, drained

1/4 cup water

1/4 cup raw unhulled sesame seeds

1 tablespoon fresh lemon juice

1 tablespoon Dr. Fuhrman's VegiZest or other no salt seasoning blend, adjusted to taste

1 teaspoon Bragg Liquid Aminos or low sodium soy sauce

1 teaspoon horseradish

1 small clove garlic, chopped

DIRECTIONS

Blend all ingredients in a high powered blender until creamy smooth.

Note: Serve with raw and lightly steamed vegetables or as a filling ingredient with a whole grain wrap or pita.

Yields: 1 cup

* *Use 1/3 cup dry beans. See cooking instructions on page*

PER SERVING: CALORIES 128; PROTEIN 6g; CARBOHYDRATES 15g; TOTAL FAT 5.5g; SATURATED FAT 0.7g; SODIUM 75mg; FIBER 4.2g; BETA-CAROTENE 307ug; VITAMIN C 5mg; CALCIUM 112mg; IRON 2.7mg; FOLATE 80ug; MAGNESIUM 52mg; ZINC 1.3mg; SELENIUM 2.1ug

SOUPS

APPLE CINNAMON BUTTERNUT SQUASH SOUP

Serves: 6

INGREDIENTS

4 cups frozen butternut squash

2 medium apples, peeled, seeded and chopped

4 cups (packed) kale, tough stems and center ribs removed and leaves chopped or frozen, chopped

1 cup chopped onion

2 tablespoons Dr. Fuhrman's Pomegranate Vinegar or other fruit flavored vinegar

5 cups carrot juice, fresh (5 pounds of carrots, juiced) or bottled

1/2 cup unsweetened soy, almond or hemp milk

1/2 cup raw cashews or 1/4 cup raw cashew butter

1 teaspoon cinnamon

1/2 teaspoon nutmeg

DIRECTIONS

Place squash, apples, kale, onion, vinegar, and carrot juice in a soup pot. Bring to a boil, then lower heat, cover, and simmer for 30 minutes or until kale is very tender.

Puree 1/2 of the soup with the milk and cashews in a food processor or high powered blender. Return blended mixture to soup pot. Add cinnamon and nutmeg.

Note: For a quick and delicious holiday breakfast, make this recipe the night before, refrigerate, and then reheat before serving.

PER SERVING: CALORIES 260; PROTEIN 8g; CARBOHYDRATES 49g; TOTAL FAT 6.6g; SATURATED FAT 1.3g; SODIUM 96mg; FIBER 6.7g; BETA-CAROTENE 26447ug; VITAMIN C 94mg; CALCIUM 180mg; IRON 3.5mg; FOLATE 64ug; MAGNESIUM 115mg; ZINC 1.5mg; SELENIUM 4.5ug

Black Forest
Cream of Mushroom Soup

Serves: 5

INGREDIENTS

2 tablespoons water

2 pounds mixed fresh mushrooms (button, shiitake, cremini) sliced 1/4" thick

2 cloves garlic, minced or pressed

2 teaspoons herbes de Provence

5 cups carrot juice fresh (5 pounds of carrots, juiced) or bottled

3 cups unsweetened hemp, soy or almond milk, divided

2 carrots, coarsely chopped

2 medium onions, chopped

3/4 cup fresh or frozen corn kernels

1 cup chopped celery

3 leeks, cut in 1/2-inch-thick rounds

1/4 cup Dr. Fuhrman's VegiZest or other no-salt seasoning, adjusted to taste

1/4 cup raw cashews

1 tablespoon fresh lemon juice

1 tablespoon chopped fresh thyme

2 teaspoons chopped fresh rosemary

3 cups cooked white beans* (northern, navy, cannellini)
or 2 (15 ounce) cans white beans, no-salt-added or low sodium, drained

5 ounces baby spinach

1/4 cup chopped fresh parsley, for garnish

DIRECTIONS

Heat the water in a large sauté pan. Water sauté the mushrooms, garlic and herbes de Provence for about 5 minutes, or until tender, adding more water if necessary to prevent from sticking. Set aside.

In a large soup pot, bring the carrot juice, 2 1/2 cups of the milk, carrots, onion, corn, celery, leeks and VegiZest to a boil. Reduce the heat and simmer until the vegetables are tender, about 30 minutes.

In a food processor or high powered blender, puree the cashews and remaining 1/2 cup milk. Add half of the soup liquid and vegetables, the lemon juice, thyme, and rosemary. Blend until smooth and creamy.

Return the pureed soup mixture to the pot. Add the beans, spinach, and sautéed mushrooms. Heat until the spinach is wilted. Garnish with parsley.

Use 1 cup dried beans. See cooking instructions on page 195.

PER SERVING: CALORIES 305; PROTEIN 18g; CARBOHYDRATES 53g; TOTAL FAT 5.1g; SATURATED FAT 0.9g; SODIUM 164mg; FIBER 11g; BETA-CAROTENE 17408ug; VITAMIN C 36mg; CALCIUM 186mg; IRON 6mg; FOLATE 188ug; MAGNESIUM 133mg; ZINC 2.4mg; SELENIUM 19.9ug

BROCCOLI LENTIL SOUP

Serves: 8

INGREDIENTS

8 cups water

2 cups carrot juice, fresh (2 pounds of carrots, juiced) or bottled

1 pound dried lentils

2 pounds plum tomatoes, chopped

4 cups chopped broccoli

2 onions, chopped

3 celery stalks, chopped

2 carrots, chopped

6 cloves garlic, minced

3 small zucchini, chopped

1 tablespoon dried oregano

1 1/2 teaspoons dried basil

1 teaspoon ground coriander

1 teaspoon ground cumin

1 teaspoon dried thyme

1 yam, peeled and chopped

3 tablespoons Dr. Fuhrman's Riesling Reserve Vinegar or balsamic vinegar

1/2 cup raw cashews or 1/4 cup raw cashew butter

DIRECTIONS

Place all ingredients except yam, vinegar and cashews in a large soup pot. Bring to a simmer and cook for 45 minutes. Add yam and simmer for an additional 15 minutes or until lentils and vegetables are tender.

Remove from heat. Add vinegar.

Remove 2 cups or more of soup and puree with the cashews in a food processor or high powered blender. Stir back into soup.

PER SERVING: CALORIES 371; PROTEIN 24g; CARBOHYDRATES 63g; TOTAL FAT 5.4g; SATURATED FAT 1g; SODIUM 84mg; FIBER 23.5g; BETA-CAROTENE 7615ug; VITAMIN C 82mg; CALCIUM 140mg; IRON 6.6mg; FOLATE 366ug; MAGNESIUM 148mg; ZINC 4mg; SELENIUM 8ug

CHUNKY SWEET POTATO STEW

Serves: 2

INGREDIENTS

1 onion, thickly sliced

2 large garlic cloves, chopped

1 1/2 cups stewed tomatoes with juice*
or 1 (15 ounce) can stewed tomatoes, no-salt-added or low sodium

1 large sweet potato, peeled, cut into 1/2 inch pieces

1/2 cup cooked garbanzo beans (chick peas) or white kidney beans

3/4 teaspoon dried rosemary

1 medium zucchini, cut into 1/2 inch thick rounds

1 teaspoon Mrs. Dash no salt seasoning

DIRECTIONS

In a sauté pan, heat 2 tablespoons water. Add the onion and water sauté about 5 minutes, until slightly softened, separating slices into rings. Add garlic and cook 1 minute. Add water as necessary to prevent from scorching.

Mix in stewed tomatoes with juice, sweet potatoes, garbanzo beans and rosemary. Bring mixture to a simmer, stirring occasionally. Cover and cook 5 minutes. Add zucchini. Cover and cook until sweet potatoes are tender, about 15 minutes, stirring occasionally. Season with Mrs. Dash.

* *To make homemade stewed tomatoes: place whole tomatoes in boiling water for 1 minute and then immediately transfer to cold water. Peel and quarter tomatoes, and place in a large saucepan. Slowly simmer over low heat for 20 to 30 minutes, stirring occasionally to prevent burning.*

PER SERVING: CALORIES 253; PROTEIN 9g; CARBOHYDRATES 50g; TOTAL FAT 3.6g; SATURATED FAT 0.6g; SODIUM 392mg; FIBER 7.9g; BETA-CAROTENE 6686ug; VITAMIN C 51mg; CALCIUM 120mg; IRON 3.3mg; FOLATE 150ug; MAGNESIUM 80mg; ZINC 1.5mg; SELENIUM 4ug

CREAMY CRUCIFEROUS CURRY

Serves: 4

INGREDIENTS

2 onions, finely diced

4 cloves garlic, minced

3 carrots, diced

3 parsnips, diced

2 cups unsweetened soy, hemp or almond milk

1 head cauliflower, cut into small florets

2 cups sliced mushrooms

1 tablespoon curry powder

1 teaspoon turmeric

1 teaspoon cumin

1 pound kale, tough stems removed, leaves chopped

1 cup frozen green peas, thawed

2 cups cooked garbanzo beans* or canned garbanzo beans, no-salt-added or low sodium, drained

1/2 cup raw cashews, chopped

DIRECTIONS

In a large stock pot over medium heat, water sauté onions, garlic, carrots and parsnips until onions are translucent (about 5 minutes).

Stir in soy milk, cauliflower, mushrooms, curry powder, turmeric, and cumin and cook for 10 minutes, covered, over medium low heat.

Stir in kale, green peas, and chick peas and continue to cook, covered for another 15 minutes or until vegetables are tender.

Top each serving with chopped cashews.

Use 2/3 cup dry beans. See cooking instructions on page 195.

PER SERVING: CALORIES 522; PROTEIN 28g; CARBOHYDRATES 82g; TOTAL FAT 13.5g; SATURATED FAT 2.1g; SODIUM 253mg; FIBER 19.1g; BETA-CAROTENE 15168ug; VITAMIN C 233mg; CALCIUM 356mg; IRON 9.5mg; FOLATE 374ug; MAGNESIUM 226mg; ZINC 4.9mg; SELENIUM 21.2ug

CREAMY ZUCCHINI SOUP

Serves: 4

INGREDIENTS

1 large onion, chopped

3 cloves garlic, chopped

2 pounds zucchini (about 5 medium), chopped

1 teaspoon dried basil

1/2 teaspoon dried thyme

1/2 teaspoon dried oregano

4 cups low sodium or no-salt-added vegetable broth

1/4 cup raw cashews or 1/8 cup raw cashew butter

4 cups baby spinach

2 cups corn kernels*

1/4 teaspoon black pepper or to taste

DIRECTIONS

Add onion, garlic, zucchini, basil, thyme, oregano and vegetable broth to a large soup pot. Bring to a boil, reduce heat and simmer for 25 minutes or until zucchini is tender.

Pour into a food processor or high powered blender (in batches, if necessary), add the cashews and blend until smooth and creamy.

Return soup to the pot, add corn and baby spinach, bring to a simmer and cook until spinach is wilted. Add water if needed to adjust consistency. Season with black pepper

* Use fresh or defrosted frozen corn kernels. If using fresh corn, steam 2 ears of corn until tender, about 7 minutes. Cut kernels from cobs with a sharp knife.

PER SERVING: CALORIES 195; PROTEIN 10g; CARBOHYDRATES 33g; TOTAL FAT 5.4g; SATURATED FAT 1.1g; SODIUM 431mg; FIBER 6.9g; BETA-CAROTENE 1981ug; VITAMIN C 72mg; CALCIUM 102mg; IRON 3.3mg; FOLATE 165ug; MAGNESIUM 105mg; ZINC 1.8mg; SELENIUM 2.7ug

DR. FUHRMAN'S FAMOUS ANTI-CANCER SOUP

Serves: 10

INGREDIENTS

1 cup dried split peas and/or beans

4 cups water

6-10 medium zucchini

5 pounds carrots, juiced (5-6 cups juice; see note)*

2 bunches celery, juiced (2 cups juice; see note)*

2 tablespoons Dr. Fuhrman's VegiZest
or other no-salt seasoning blend such as Mrs. Dash, adjusted to taste

4 medium onions, chopped

3 leek stalks, coarsely chopped

2 bunches kale, collard greens or other greens,
tough stems and center ribs removed and leaves chopped

1 cup raw cashews

2 1/2 cups chopped fresh mushrooms (shiitake, cremini and/or white)

DIRECTIONS

Place the beans and water in a very large pot over low heat. Bring to a boil, reduce heat and simmer. Add the zucchini whole to the pot. Add the carrot juice, celery juice and VegiZest.

Put the onions, leeks and kale in a blender and blend with a little bit of the soup liquid. Pour this mixture into the soup pot.

Remove the softened zucchini with tongs and blend them in the blender with the cashews until creamy. Pour this mixture back into the soup pot. Add the mushrooms and continue to simmer the beans until soft, about 2 hours total cooking time.

* *Freshly juiced organic carrots and celery will maximize the flavor of this soup.*

PER SERVING: CALORIES 322; PROTEIN 16g; CARBOHYDRATES 56g; TOTAL FAT 7.4g; SATURATED FAT 1.3g; SODIUM 130mg; FIBER 12g; BETA-CAROTENE 24498ug; VITAMIN C 165mg; CALCIUM 236mg; IRON 5.6mg; FOLATE 174ug; MAGNESIUM 162mg; ZINC 2.8mg; SELENIUM 7.8ug

EASY THREE BEAN VEGETABLE CHILI

Serves: 6

INGREDIENTS

1 pound firm tofu, frozen, then defrosted

2 tablespoons chili powder, or to taste

1 teaspoon cumin

10 ounces frozen onions

3 cups frozen broccoli, thawed and finely chopped

3 cups frozen cauliflower, thawed and finely chopped

3 cloves garlic, chopped

1 1/2 cups cooked pinto beans* or 1 (15 ounce) can pinto beans, no-salt-added or low sodium, drained

1 1/2 cups cooked black beans* or 1 (15 ounce) can black beans, no-salt-added or low sodium, drained

1 1/2 cups cooked red beans* or 1 (15 ounce) can red beans, no-salt-added or low sodium, drained

1 (28 ounce can) diced tomatoes, no-salt-added or low sodium

1 (4 ounce can) chopped mild green chilis

2 1/2 cups fresh or frozen corn kernels

2 large zucchini, finely chopped

DIRECTIONS

Squeeze excess water out of thawed tofu and crumble. Place the crumbled tofu, chili powder and cumin in a soup pot and quickly brown. Add the remaining ingredients and simmer, covered, for 2 hours.

* Use 1/2 cup of each type of dried bean. See cooking instructions on page 195.

PER SERVING: CALORIES 384; PROTEIN 21g; CARBOHYDRATES 75g; TOTAL FAT 3.7g; SATURATED FAT 0.5g; SODIUM 824mg; FIBER 21.9g; BETA-CAROTENE 1011ug; VITAMIN C 116mg; CALCIUM 252mg; IRON 7.2mg; FOLATE 318ug; MAGNESIUM 162mg; ZINC 3.1mg; SELENIUM 14.2ug

FRENCH MINTED PEA SOUP

Serves: 3

INGREDIENTS

10 ounces frozen green peas

1 small onion, chopped

1 clove garlic, chopped

1 bunch fresh mint leaves (save a few leaves for garnish)

3 tablespoons Dr. Fuhrman's VegiZest, or other no salt soup base seasoning, adjusted to taste

3 cups water

3 dates, pitted

1/2 cup raw cashews or 1/4 cup raw cashew butter

1/2 tablespoon Spike no salt seasoning, or other no salt seasoning, to taste

4 teaspoons fresh lemon juice

4 cups shredded romaine lettuce or chopped baby spinach

2 tablespoons fresh snipped chives

DIRECTIONS

Simmer peas, onions, garlic, mint and VegiZest in water for about 7 minutes.

Pour pea mixture into a high powered blender or food processor. Add remaining ingredients except for the lettuce and chives. Blend until smooth and creamy.

Add lettuce or spinach and let it wilt in hot liquid.

Pour into bowls and garnish with chives and mint leaves.

PER SERVING: CALORIES 301; PROTEIN 14g; CARBOHYDRATES 44g; TOTAL FAT 10.4g; SATURATED FAT 1.8g; SODIUM 180mg; FIBER 10.1g; BETA-CAROTENE 5661ug; VITAMIN C 54mg; CALCIUM 150mg; IRON 8.4mg; FOLATE 219ug; MAGNESIUM 134mg; ZINC 2.7mg; SELENIUM 7.2ug

GOLDEN AUSTRIAN CAULIFLOWER CREAM SOUP

Serves: 4

INGREDIENTS

1 head cauliflower, cut into pieces

3 carrots, coarsely chopped

1 cup coarsely chopped celery

2 leeks, coarsely chopped

2 cloves garlic, minced

2 tablespoons Dr. Fuhrman's VegiZest
or other no salt seasoning blend such as Mrs. Dash, adjusted to taste

2 cups carrot juice, fresh (2 pounds of carrots juiced) or bottled

4 cups water

1/2 teaspoon nutmeg

1 cup raw cashews or 1/2 cup raw cashew butter

5 cups chopped kale leaves or baby spinach

DIRECTIONS

Place all the ingredients except the cashews and kale in a pot. Cover and simmer for 15 minutes or until the vegetables are just tender. Steam the kale until tender. If you are using spinach there is no need to steam it; it will wilt in the hot soup.

In a food processor or high powered blender, blend two-thirds of the soup liquid and vegetables with the cashews until smooth and creamy. Return to the pot and stir in the steamed kale (or raw spinach).

PER SERVING: CALORIES 354; PROTEIN 13g; CARBOHYDRATES 46g; TOTAL FAT 16.7g; SATURATED FAT 3.4g; SODIUM 202mg; FIBER 9.1g; BETA-CAROTENE 18003ug; VITAMIN C 102mg; CALCIUM 176mg; IRON 5.8mg; FOLATE 233ug; MAGNESIUM 182mg; ZINC 3mg; SELENIUM 6.8ug

High Cruciferous Vegetable Stew

Serves: 10

INGREDIENTS

4 cups water

2 1/2 cups carrot juice, fresh (2 1/2 pounds of carrots, juiced) or bottled

1/2 cup dried split peas

1/2 cup dried lentils

1/2 cup adzuki beans, soaked overnight

1 bunch kale, tough stems and center ribs removed
and leaves coarsely chopped

1 bunch collard greens, tough stems and center ribs removed
and leaves coarsely chopped

1 head broccoli, cut into florets

8 ounces shiitake mushrooms, cut in half

3 celery stalks, cut into 1-inch pieces

3 leeks, coarsely chopped

3 carrots, cut into 1-inch pieces

3 parsnips, cut into 1-inch pieces

3 medium onions, chopped

4 medium zucchini, cubed

4 cloves garlic, chopped

1 (28-ounce) can chopped tomatoes, no-salt-added or low sodium

1/4 cup Dr. Fuhrman's VegiZest or other
no-salt seasoning blend, adjusted to taste

2 tablespoons Mrs. Dash seasoning

1/4 cup chopped fresh parsley

1 cup broccoli sprouts

DIRECTIONS

Place all the ingredients except the parsley and sprouts in a very large soup pot. Cover and bring to a simmer, cooking until the adzuki beans are tender, about 1 1/2 hours.

In a food processor or high powered blender, blend one-quarter of the soup until smooth. Return to the soup pot and stir in the parsley and broccoli sprouts.

PER SERVING: CALORIES 321; PROTEIN 19g; CARBOHYDRATES 67g; TOTAL FAT 1.7g; SATURATED FAT 0.3g; SODIUM 171mg; FIBER 15.8g; BETA-CAROTENE 28077ug; VITAMIN C 154mg; CALCIUM 217mg; IRON 5.6mg; FOLATE 294ug; MAGNESIUM 135mg; ZINC 2.8mg; SELENIUM 7.8ug

QUICK AND CREAMY VEGETABLE BEAN SOUP

Serves: 8

INGREDIENTS

4 cups vegetable broth, no-salt-added or low sodium

2 cups frozen broccoli florets

2 cups frozen chopped spinach

2 cups carrot juice, fresh (2 pounds of carrots, juiced) or bottled

1 cup chopped onions

4 1/2 cups cooked cannellini beans*
or 3 (15 ounce) cans cannellini beans, no-salt-added or low sodium, drained

3 fresh tomatoes, chopped

1 bunch fresh basil, chopped

4 tablespoons Dr. Fuhrman's VegiZest or other no salt seasoning blend, adjusted to taste

1 teaspoon garlic powder

1/2 teaspoon dried basil

1/2 teaspoon dried oregano

1/2 cup raw cashew nuts or 1/4 cup raw cashew butter

1/4 cup pine nuts

DIRECTIONS

In soup pot, combine all ingredients, except cashews and pine nuts. Cover and simmer for 30-40 minutes.

In high powered blender, blend 1/4 of soup mixture with cashew nuts. Add back to soup pot.

Serve with pine nuts sprinkled on top.

* Use 1 1/2 cups dried beans. See cooking instructions on page 195.

PER SERVING: CALORIES 355; PROTEIN 20g; CARBOHYDRATES 57g; TOTAL FAT 8.7g; SATURATED FAT 1.3g; SODIUM 111mg; FIBER 11.5g; BETA-CAROTENE 9623ug; VITAMIN C 81mg; CALCIUM 228mg; IRON 8mg; FOLATE 198ug; MAGNESIUM 167mg; ZINC 3.1mg; SELENIUM 8.5ug

SOUTHWEST VEGETABLE STEW

Serves: 3

INGREDIENTS

1 large potato, cut into small pieces

1/2 medium green bell pepper, chopped

1/2 medium red bell pepper, chopped

1/2 medium onion, chopped

1-2 small jalapeno peppers, seeded and chopped

2 large cloves garlic, chopped

1 1/2 tablespoons chili powder

1 (14-ounce) can chopped tomatoes, no-salt-added or low sodium

1 cup fresh or frozen corn

1 1/2 cups cooked black cooked black beans*
or 1 (15 ounce) can black beans, no-salt-added or low sodium, drained

2 tablespoons chopped fresh cilantro

DIRECTIONS

Place potatoes in a pot and cover with water. Simmer for about 8 minutes until tender. Drain and set aside.

Heat 1/8 cup water in a large saucepan over medium heat. Add green and red peppers, onions, jalapenos, and garlic and water sauté for 2 minutes. Add chili powder and stir for one minute. Add tomatoes, corn, beans, cilantro, and reserved potatoes. Simmer until potatoes are very tender, stirring occasionally, for about 20 minutes.

* Use 1/2 cup dry beans. See cooking instructions on page 195.

PER SERVING: CALORIES 364; PROTEIN 18g; CARBOHYDRATES 71g; TOTAL FAT 3.8g; SATURATED FAT 0.7g; SODIUM 71mg; FIBER 19.3g; BETA-CAROTENE 1196ug; VITAMIN C 80mg; CALCIUM 121mg; IRON 6mg; FOLATE 285ug; MAGNESIUM 157mg; ZINC 2.4mg; SELENIUM 3.3ug

TOMATO BISQUE

Serves: 4

INGREDIENTS

3 cups carrot juice, fresh (about 3 pounds of carrots, juiced) or bottled

1 1/2 pounds fresh chopped tomatoes
or 1 (28 ounce) can whole tomatoes, no-salt-added
or low sodium (San Marzano variety, if possible)

1/4 cup unsalted, unsulfured sun-dried tomatoes, chopped

2 celery stalks, chopped

1 small onion, chopped

1 leek, chopped

1 large shallot, chopped

3 cloves garlic, chopped

2 tablespoons Dr. Fuhrman's MatoZest
or other no salt seasoning blend, adjusted to taste

1 teaspoon dried thyme, crumbled

1 small bay leaf

1/2 cup raw cashews or 1/4 cup raw cashew butter

1/4 cup chopped fresh basil

5 ounces baby spinach

DIRECTIONS

In a large saucepan, add all ingredients except the cashews, basil and spinach. Simmer for 30 minutes. Discard the bay leaf.

Remove 2 cups of the vegetables with a slotted spoon and set aside. Puree the remaining soup with the cashews in a food processor or high powered blender until smooth. Return the pureed soup along with the reserved vegetables to the pot. Stir in the basil and spinach and heat until spinach is wilted.

PER SERVING: CALORIES 254; PROTEIN 14g; CARBOHYDRATES 40g; TOTAL FAT 8.9g; SATURATED FAT 1.7g; SODIUM 203mg; FIBER 6.3g; BETA-CAROTENE 20201ug; VITAMIN C 57mg; CALCIUM 141mg; IRON 4.4mg; FOLATE 143ug; MAGNESIUM 133mg; ZINC 1.8mg; SELENIUM 4.2ug

TUSCAN BEANS AND GREENS SOUP

Serves: 6

INGREDIENTS

1 cup unsulfured, unsalted sun-dried tomatoes

1/2 cup unsweetened soy, hemp or almond milk

1 cup chopped onions

2 cloves garlic, minced

1 teaspoon dried basil

1 teaspoon dried oregano

1/2 teaspoon dried crushed rosemary

1 1/2 cups cooked white beans*
or 1 (15 ounce) can white beans, no-salt-added or low sodium, drained

1 1/2 cups diced tomatoes, or 1 (15 ounce) can no-salt-added or low
sodium, with liquid

3 cups no-salt-added or low sodium vegetable broth

1 cup water

6 cups chopped collard greens

1 tablespoon Dr. Fuhrman's Black Fig Vinegar or balsamic vinegar

1/2 teaspoon freshly ground black pepper

1 tablespoon Dr. Fuhrman's MatoZest
or other no salt seasoning blend, adjusted to taste

DIRECTIONS

Soak the sun-dried tomatoes in soy milk for one hour to soften. Drain,
reserving soy milk. Chop tomatoes finely and set aside.

Heat 1/8 cup water over medium heat. Add onions and garlic and water saute
for 5 minutes, until onions are soft. If necessary, add more water to keep from
sticking. Stir in sun-dried tomatoes, soy milk, basil, oregano, and rosemary.

Add the beans, diced tomatoes, vegetable broth and water. Bring to a boil.
Add the greens, lower heat and simmer for about 20 minutes.

Before serving, stir in the vinegar, black pepper and MatoZest

* Use 1/2 cup dry beans. See cooking instructions on page 195.

PER SERVING: CALORIES 182; PROTEIN 15g; CARBOHYDRATES 32g; TOTAL FAT 2.4g; SATURATED FAT 0.5g;
SODIUM 279mg; FIBER 11.1g; BETA-CAROTENE 9693ug; VITAMIN C 48mg; CALCIUM 344mg; IRON 5.1mg;
FOLATE 245ug; MAGNESIUM 95mg; ZINC 1.4mg; SELENIUM 4.5ug

MAIN DISHES

ACORN SQUASH SUPREME

Serves: 2

INGREDIENTS

1 large acorn squash

1/4 cup dried unsulfured apricots,
soaked in just enough water to almost cover until soft, then diced

1 1/2 cups pineapple, chopped

2 tablespoons raisins

2 tablespoons chopped raw cashews

cinnamon

DIRECTIONS

Cut squash in half, remove seeds, and bake face down in 1/2 inch of water for 45 minutes at 350° F.

Meanwhile, combine the apricots and soaking liquid, pineapple, raisins, and cashews.

After the squash has cooked, scoop the fruit/nut mixture into the squash's center. Place in pan and cover loosely with aluminum foil. Bake for an additional 30 minutes. Sprinkle with cinnamon, then put it back in the oven for 5 more minutes.

PER SERVING: CALORIES 257; PROTEIN 4g; CARBOHYDRATES 57g; TOTAL FAT 4.4g; SATURATED FAT 0.8g; SODIUM 12mg; FIBER 6.6g; BETA-CAROTENE 865ug; VITAMIN C 66mg; CALCIUM 104mg; IRON 3mg; FOLATE 62ug; MAGNESIUM 113mg; ZINC 1mg; SELENIUM 2.6ug

ARTICHOKE LENTIL LOAF

Serves: 6

INGREDIENTS

2 large artichokes, rinsed or 6 frozen artichoke hearts, thawed and mashed

1/2 cup diced onion

2 cloves garlic, minced

3 cups finely chopped mushrooms

1/4 cup diced celery

2 tablespoons minced parsley

1/2 teaspoon poultry seasoning

1 1/2 cups cooked lentils
or 1 (15 ounce) can lentils, no-salt-added or low sodium, rinsed and drained

1/3 cup finely chopped raw pecans

1/4 cup rolled oats

1/4 cup tomato paste (plus extra reserved for top of loaf)

2 tablespoons arrowroot powder (or whole wheat flour)

2 tablespoons MatoZest or other no salt seasoning blend, adjusted to taste

freshly ground black pepper, to taste

DIRECTIONS

Preheat oven to 350° F.

If using fresh artichokes, slice one inch off the top of each artichoke. Cut off the very bottom of the stem, but keep the stems attached. Slice artichokes in half, lengthwise. Place them in a steamer basket over several inches of water. Bring water to a boil, cover and steam for 40 minutes. Set artichokes aside until cool enough to handle. Scoop out and discard the fibrous choke from the center of each artichoke. Remove the hearts and transfer to a bowl. Mash lightly. Scrape off the bottom one third of each leaf and add to mashed hearts. Carefully scrape out the tender insides of the stems to use as well.

In a sauté pan, heat one tablespoon of water or vegetable broth. Add onion and garlic and sauté for 5 minutes. Add mushrooms, cover and cook until mushrooms are tender. Add celery, parsley and poultry seasoning. Sauté another 5 minutes, adding more water if needed to prevent sticking.

Place the sautéed vegetables in a bowl and add the lentils, 1 cup of mashed artichokes, pecans, rolled oats, tomato paste, arrowroot powder, MatoZest and black pepper. Stir well to combine.

Lightly rub a loaf pan with minimal amount of oil. Fill the loaf pan with lentil mixture and press down evenly. Spread a 1/8 inch layer of reserved tomato paste over top. Bake for 1 hour. Remove from oven and let stand at room temperature for 30 minutes before slicing and serving.

Makes 1 loaf

PER SERVING: CALORIES 189; PROTEIN 9g; CARBOHYDRATES 29g; TOTAL FAT 5.3g; SATURATED FAT 0.5g; SODIUM 146mg; FIBER 8.7g; BETA-CAROTENE 622ug; VITAMIN C 13mg; CALCIUM 51mg; IRON 3.6mg; FOLATE 130ug; MAGNESIUM 73mg; ZINC 1.7mg; SELENIUM 8.6ug

ASIAN VEGETABLE STIR FRY

Serves: 4

INGREDIENTS

14 ounces extra firm tofu, cubed

1 teaspoon Bragg Liquid Aminos or low sodium soy sauce

1/4 teaspoon crushed red pepper flakes

2 tablespoons Spike no salt seasoning (or other no-salt seasoning blend adjusted to taste)

1/2 cup brown rice

1/4 cup unhulled sesame seeds

FOR THE SAUCE:

1/4 cup unsulfured dried apricots soaked in 1/2 cup water to cover overnight

1/4 cup unsalted natural peanut butter or raw cashew butter

2 tablespoons fresh chopped ginger

4 cloves garlic, chopped

4 teaspoons Dr. Fuhrman's VegiZest or other no-salt seasoning blend, adjusted to taste

1/4 cup Dr. Fuhrman's Black Fig vinegar or balsamic vinegar

1 teaspoon arrowroot powder

1/4 teaspoon crushed red pepper flakes

FOR THE VEGETABLES:

2 tablespoons water

1 medium onion, cut into wedges and separated into 1-inch strips

4 cups small broccoli florets

2 medium carrots, cut diagonally into 1/3 inch pieces

4 medium red bell peppers, seeded and cut into 1 inch squares

1 cup sugar snap peas or snow peas, strings removed

2 cups bok choy, cut in bite-sized pieces

3 cups fresh mushrooms (shiitake, porcini and/or cremini) , stems removed

1 pound fresh spinach

1/2 cup coarsely chopped raw cashews

1 1/4 pounds romaine lettuce, shredded

DIRECTIONS

Marinate the tofu for 30 minutes in the liquid aminos, red pepper flakes and Spike. While the tofu marinates, combine rice and 1 1/4 cups water in a saucepan. Bring to a boil. Reduce heat and cover. Simmer 30 minutes or until water is absorbed and rice is tender. Set aside.

Preheat the oven to 350° F. Toss the marinated tofu with the sesame seeds. Bake the sesame-coated tofu in a nonstick baking pan for 30 minutes.

To make the sauce, place the soaked apricots with the soaking liquid, peanut butter, ginger, garlic, VegiZest, vinegar, arrowroot powder, and red pepper flakes in a food processor or high powered blender and blend until smooth. Transfer to a small bowl and set aside.

Heat water in a large pan and water sauté the onion, broccoli, carrots, bell peppers, and peas for 5 minutes, adding more water as necessary to keep vegetables from scorching. Add the bok choy and mushrooms, cover, and simmer until the vegetables are just tender. Remove the cover and cook off most of the water. Add the spinach and toss until wilted.

Add the sauce and stir until all the vegetables are glazed and the sauce is hot and bubbly, about 1 minute. Mix in the cashews and baked tofu. Serve the stir fry over the shredded lettuce along with 1/4 cup rice per person.

Variation: Stir-fry beans or small pieces of chicken breast or shrimp with the vegetables.

PER SERVING: CALORIES 386; PROTEIN 17g; CARBOHYDRATES 51g; TOTAL FAT 16.2g; SATURATED FAT 2.9g; SODIUM 190mg; FIBER 11g; BETA-CAROTENE 11814ug; VITAMIN C 223mg; CALCIUM 319mg; IRON 7.9mg; FOLATE 433ug; MAGNESIUM 220mg; ZINC 3.6mg; SELENIUM 19.5ug

BEAN ENCHILADAS

Serves: 6

INGREDIENTS

1 medium green bell pepper, seeded and chopped

1/2 cup sliced onion

8 ounces no-salt-added or low sodium tomato sauce, divided

2 cups cooked pinto or black beans* or canned beans,
no-salt-added or low sodium, drained

1 cup frozen corn kernels

1 tablespoon chili powder

1 teaspoon ground cumin

1 teaspoon onion powder

1/8 teaspoon cayenne pepper, if desired

1 tablespoon chopped fresh cilantro

6 corn tortillas

DIRECTIONS

Sauté the green pepper and onion in 2 tablespoons of the tomato sauce until tender. Stir in the remaining tomato sauce, beans, corn, chili powder, cumin, onion powder, cilantro and cayenne (if using). Simmer for 5 minutes. Spoon about 1/4 cup of the bean mixture on each tortilla and roll up. Serve as is or bake for 15 minutes in a 375° F oven.

* *Use 2/3 cup dried beans. See cooking instructions on page 195.*

PER SERVING: CALORIES 187; PROTEIN 8g; CARBOHYDRATES 37g; TOTAL FAT 1.7g; SATURATED FAT 0.3g;
SODIUM 33mg; FIBER 9g; BETA-CAROTENE 351ug; VITAMIN C 25mg; CALCIUM 57mg; IRON 2.2mg;
FOLATE 107ug; MAGNESIUM 77mg; ZINC 1.3mg; SELENIUM 2.9ug

BETTER BURGERS

Serves: 8

INGREDIENTS

1 1/2 cups old fashioned rolled oats

1 cup ground walnuts

1 cup water

1/4 cup tomato paste

1/4 cup Dr. Fuhrman's MatoZest or
other no salt seasoning blend, adjusted to taste

1 cup diced onion

3 cloves garlic, minced

6 cups finely minced mushrooms

2 teaspoons dried basil

1/2 teaspoon dried oregano

2 tablespoons fresh parsley, minced

freshly ground pepper, to taste

2/3 cup frozen chopped spinach, thawed

DIRECTIONS

Preheat oven to 350° F.

Combine rolled oats and ground walnuts in a bowl. Set aside.

In a small saucepan, whisk together water, tomato paste and MatoZest. Heat over medium-high heat until boiling. Pour over rolled oats and walnuts. Stir well and set aside.

Heat 2 tablespoons water in a sauté pan and add onion and garlic. Saute until onion is translucent. Add mushrooms, basil, oregano, parsley and black pepper and additional water if needed, to prevent sticking. Cover and cook for 5 minutes, or until mushrooms are tender.

In a large bowl, combine sautéed onions and mushrooms, rolled oat/walnut mixture and spinach. Stir well to combine. With wet hands, shape 1/3 cup of mixture into a well-formed burger. Place on a lightly oiled baking sheet and repeat with remaining mixture. Bake for 15 minutes. Turn burgers to bake the other side for another 15 minutes.

Remove from oven and cool slightly. Serve on small whole grain hamburger buns or whole grain pita bread halves. Top with thin sliced, raw red onion and low sodium ketchup.

Makes 12 burgers

PER SERVING: CALORIES 199; PROTEIN 9g; CARBOHYDRATES 21g; TOTAL FAT 11.1g; SATURATED FAT 1.1g; SODIUM 101mg; FIBER 4.4g; BETA-CAROTENE 1642ug; VITAMIN C 12mg; CALCIUM 50mg; IRON 2.5mg; FOLATE 55ug; MAGNESIUM 86mg; ZINC 1.5mg; SELENIUM 14.1ug

BLACK BEAN LETTUCE BUNDLES

Serves: 4

INGREDIENTS

2 cups cooked black beans* or canned black beans, no-salt-added or low sodium, drained

1/2 large ripe avocado, peeled, pitted and mashed

1/2 medium green bell pepper, seeded and chopped

3 green onions, chopped

1/3 cup chopped fresh cilantro

1/3 cup mild, no-salt-added or low sodium salsa

2 tablespoons fresh lime juice

1 clove garlic, minced

1 teaspoon ground cumin

8 large romaine lettuce leaves

DIRECTIONS

In a bowl, mash the beans and avocado together with a fork until well blended and only slightly chunky. Add all the remaining ingredients except the lettuce and mix.

Place approximately 1/4 cup of the mixture in the center of each lettuce leaf and roll up like a burrito.

* Use 2/3 cups dried beans. See cooking instructions on page 195.

PER SERVING: CALORIES 171; PROTEIN 10g; CARBOHYDRATES 27g; TOTAL FAT 4.1g; SATURATED FAT 0.6g; SODIUM 13mg; FIBER 11g; BETA-CAROTENE 2470ug; VITAMIN C 26mg; CALCIUM 63mg; IRON 2.8mg; FOLATE 231ug; MAGNESIUM 80mg; ZINC 1.3mg; SELENIUM 1.6ug

BRAISED BOK CHOY

Serves: 2

INGREDIENTS

8 baby bok choy or 3 regular bok choy

1 teaspoon Bragg Liquid Aminos or low sodium soy sauce

2 cups coarsely chopped shiitake mushrooms

2 large cloves garlic, chopped

1 tablespoon unhulled sesame seeds, lightly toasted *

DIRECTIONS

Cover bottom of large skillet with 1/2 inch water. Add bok choy (cut baby bok choy in half lengthwise or cut regular bok choy into chunks).

Drizzle with liquid aminos. Cover and cook on high heat until bok choy is tender, about 6 minutes.

Remove bok choy and add mushrooms and garlic to the liquid.

Simmer mushrooms and garlic until tender. Pour over bok choy. Top with toasted sesame seeds.

Lightly toast sesame seeds in a pan over medium heat for 3 minutes, shaking pan frequently.

PER SERVING: CALORIES 53; PROTEIN 5g; CARBOHYDRATES 4g; TOTAL FAT 1.7g; SATURATED FAT 0.2g; CHOLESTEROL 0.1mg; SODIUM 244mg; FIBER 3.5g; VITAMIN C 42mg; CALCIUM 157mg; IRON 1.8mg; FOLATE 83ug; MAGNESIUM 39mg; ZINC 0.8mg; SELENIUM 1.6ug

BRAISED KALE AND SQUASH WITH PUMPKIN SEEDS

Serves: 6

INGREDIENTS

2 bunches kale, tough stems and center ribs removed and leaves chopped

1 medium butternut squash or small pumpkin, peeled, seeded and cubed

2 medium red onions, coarsely chopped

6 cloves garlic, sliced

2 tablespoons Dr. Fuhrman's VegiZest
or other no salt seasoning blend, adjusted to taste

2/3 cup water

3 tablespoons Dr. Fuhrman's Black Fig Vinegar or balsamic vinegar

1 cup raw pumpkin seeds or sunflower seeds, lightly toasted

DIRECTIONS

Place kale, squash, onion, garlic, and VegiZest in a large pot with water. Cover and steam over low heat for 20 minutes or until kale and squash are tender.

Add vinegar and toss. Serve sprinkled with lightly toasted pumpkin or sunflower seeds.

Note: Toast seeds in oven at 300° F for 4 minutes, or until lightly toasted.

PER SERVING: CALORIES 269; PROTEIN 10g; CARBOHYDRATES 36g; TOTAL FAT 12.4g; SATURATED FAT 1.3g; SODIUM 45mg; FIBER 7.4g; BETA-CAROTENE 11669ug; VITAMIN C 97mg; CALCIUM 186mg; IRON 4mg; FOLATE 119ug; MAGNESIUM 163mg; ZINC 1.8mg; SELENIUM 16.1ug

BROCCOLI FRA DIAVLO

Serves: 2

INGREDIENTS

5 cups fresh broccoli florets

4 cloves garlic, chopped

1 1/2 cups diced fresh tomatoes
or 1 (15 ounce) can no-salt-added diced tomatoes

1 cup low sodium or no-salt-added tomato or pasta sauce

1 dash dried hot pepper flakes

1-2 teaspoons no-salt-added Italian seasoning

1/4 cup nutritional yeast

DIRECTIONS

Steam broccoli until tender.

In large saucepan over medium heat, sauté garlic in 1/4 cup water for 3-4 minutes. Add tomatoes, tomato sauce, hot pepper flakes, and Italian seasoning to taste. Simmer 10 minutes.

Stir in broccoli and nutritional yeast.

PER SERVING: CALORIES 209; PROTEIN 19g; CARBOHYDRATES 38g; TOTAL FAT 1.5g; SATURATED FAT 0.2g; SODIUM 116mg; FIBER 15g; BETA-CAROTENE 1712ug; VITAMIN C 238mg; CALCIUM 194mg; IRON 6.2mg; FOLATE 803ug; MAGNESIUM 126mg; ZINC 2.8mg; SELENIUM 7.3ug

California Creamed Kale

Serves: 4

INGREDIENTS

2 bunches kale, leaves removed from tough stems and chopped

1 cup raw cashews or 1/2 cup raw cashew butter

1 cup unsweetened soy, hemp or almond milk

4 tablespoons onion flakes

1 tablespoon Dr. Fuhrman's VegiZest
or other no-salt seasoning blend, adjusted to taste

DIRECTIONS

Place kale in a large steamer pot. Steam 10-20 minutes until soft.

Meanwhile, place remaining ingredients in a high-powered blender and blend until smooth.

Place kale in colander and press to remove the excess water. In a bowl, coarsely chop and mix kale with the cream sauce.

Note: Sauce may be used with broccoli, spinach, or other steamed vegetables.

PER SERVING: CALORIES 269; PROTEIN 12g; CARBOHYDRATES 25g; TOTAL FAT 15.9g;
SATURATED FAT 2.7g; SODIUM 78mg; FIBER 3.7g; BETA-CAROTENE 7060ug; VITAMIN C 90mg;
CALCIUM 143mg; IRON 4.3mg; FOLATE 47ug; MAGNESIUM 139mg; ZINC 2.6mg; SELENIUM 10.2ug

Cauliflower, Spinach Mashed "Potatoes"

Serves: 4

INGREDIENTS

6 cups fresh or frozen cauliflower florets

4 cloves garlic, sliced

10 ounces fresh spinach

1/2 cup raw cashew butter

soy, almond or hemp milk, if needed to thin

2 tablespoons Dr. Fuhrman's VegiZest
or other no salt seasoning blend, adjusted to taste

1/4 teaspoon nutmeg

DIRECTIONS

Steam cauliflower and garlic about 8 to 10 minutes or until tender. Drain and press out as much water as possible in strainer.

Place spinach in steamer, steam until just wilted and set aside.

Process cauliflower, garlic, and cashew butter in a food processor until creamy and smooth. If necessary, add soy milk to adjust consistency

Add VegiZest and nutmeg. Mix in wilted spinach.

PER SERVING: CALORIES 164; PROTEIN 9g; CARBOHYDRATES 18g; TOTAL FAT 8.5g; SATURATED FAT 1.7g; SODIUM 124mg; FIBER 5.7g; BETA-CAROTENE 4599ug; VITAMIN C 93mg; CALCIUM 116mg; IRON 3.8mg; FOLATE 234ug; MAGNESIUM 121mg; ZINC 1.7mg; SELENIUM 3.9ug

CREAMED FOREST KALE OVER WILD RICE

Serves: 5

INGREDIENTS

2 bunches kale, tough stems and center ribs removed
and leaves coarsely chopped

2 cups sliced shiitake mushrooms

1 medium onion, chopped

2 cups fresh or frozen peas

3/4 cup raw cashews

3/4 cup unsweetened hemp, soy or almond milk

1/4 cup onion flakes

2 cups cooked wild rice

3 tablespoons raw unhulled sesame seeds

DIRECTIONS

In a large covered skillet, water sauté the kale, mushrooms, onion, and peas over medium heat, until kale is tender, about 10 minutes. Stir occasionally and add water as needed.

Meanwhile, blend the cashews, milk and onion flakes in a food processor or high powered blender until smooth and creamy.

Stir cashew cream sauce into kale mixture.

Serve over wild rice, topped with sesame seeds.

PER SERVING: CALORIES 338; PROTEIN 15g; CARBOHYDRATES 44g; TOTAL FAT 13.9g; SATURATED FAT 2.5g; SODIUM 118mg; FIBER 7.6g; BETA-CAROTENE 6071ug; VITAMIN C 84mg; CALCIUM 183mg; IRON 5mg; FOLATE 106ug; MAGNESIUM 145mg; ZINC 3.6mg; SELENIUM 10.3ug

CREMINI RATATOUILLE

Serves: 2

INGREDIENTS

1 medium onion, thinly sliced

2 garlic cloves, chopped

2 large tomatoes, chopped or 1 (15 ounce) can no-salt-added diced tomatos

1 medium eggplant, cut into 1 inch dice

1 medium zucchini, sliced crosswise 1 inch thick

10 ounces cremini or other mushrooms, sliced

1 medium red pepper, cut into 1 inch pieces

1 teaspoon oregano

1 teaspoon basil

pepper, to taste

DIRECTIONS

Heat 1/8 cup water in a large deep skillet. Water sauté the onion until softened, about 3 minutes. Add the garlic and cook for 1 minute, adding more water as necessary to keep from scorching. Reduce the heat to moderately low and add the tomatoes, eggplant, zucchini, mushrooms, red pepper and spices. Cover and cook, stirring occasionally until vegetables are very tender, about 1 hour.

Serve warm or at room temperature.

PER SERVING: CALORIES 90; PROTEIN 7g; CARBOHYDRATES 19g; TOTAL FAT 0.9g; SATURATED FAT 0.2g; SODIUM 17mg; FIBER 7.9g; BETA-CAROTENE 863ug; VITAMIN C 61mg; CALCIUM 45mg; IRON 1.4mg; FOLATE 85ug; MAGNESIUM 49mg; ZINC 1mg; SELENIUM 7.5ug

COLLARD DIJON WRAP UPS

Serves: 2

INGREDIENTS

2 teaspoons Dijon mustard

2 pitted prunes, soaked until soft or overnight

2 teaspoons red wine vinegar

2 tablespoons shredded carrots

2 tablespoons shredded cucumber

1/4 cup chopped red onion

1/4 cup chopped green or red bell pepper

1/2 ripe avocado, peeled, pitted and cut into 4 slices

4 slices tomato

2 large collard leaves, thick stem removed

2 medium romaine leaves

DIRECTIONS

Combine the Dijon mustard, prunes, and red wine vinegar in a medium bowl and mash with a fork. Stir in carrots, cucumber, red onion and pepper.

Lay out a large collard leaf and place a romaine leaf on top of it. Top with half of the mustard/vegetable mixture and 2 slices of tomato and avocado. Roll like a burrito.

PER SERVING: CALORIES 150; PROTEIN 4g; CARBOHYDRATES 18g; TOTAL FAT 8.0g; SATURATED FAT 1.5g; SODIUM 136mg; FIBER 7.3g; BETA-CAROTENE 2816ug; VITAMIN C 56mg; CALCIUM 58mg; IRON 0.8mg; FOLATE 113ug; MAGNESIUM 36mg; ZINC 0.6mg; SELENIUM 0.5ug

CUBAN BLACK BEANS

Serves: 6

INGREDIENTS

1 cup chopped onion

3/4 cup chopped green bell pepper

2 cups no-salt-added or low sodium tomato juice

4 1/4 cups cooked black beans*
or 3 (15 ounce) cans black beans, no-salt-added or low sodium, drained

1 1/2 cups chopped tomatoes
or 1 (14 ounce) can no-salt-added or low sodium chopped tomatoes

1 cup no-salt-added tomato sauce

3 cloves garlic, minced

1 tablespoon Dr. Fuhrman's VegiZest
or other no salt seasoning blend, adjusted to taste

1 teaspoon cumin

1/2 teaspoon garlic powder

1/4 teaspoon black pepper

DIRECTIONS

Heat 1 tablespoons water in a large pan and water sauté onions and peppers until tender. Add tomato juice and next 8 ingredients; bring to a boil. Cover, reduce heat, and simmer 20 to 25 minutes or until vegetables are tender.

* Use 1 1/2 cups dry beans. See cooking instructions on page 195.

PER SERVING: CALORIES 255; PROTEIN 15g; CARBOHYDRATES 46g; TOTAL FAT 3g; SATURATED FAT 0.5g;
SODIUM 82mg; FIBER 14g; BETA-CAROTENE 1259ug; VITAMIN C 51mg; CALCIUM 73mg; IRON 3.6mg;
FOLATE 218ug; MAGNESIUM 114mg; ZINC 1.8mg; SELENIUM 2.8ug

EGGPLANT ROLL UPS

Serves: 6

INGREDIENTS

2 large eggplants, peeled and sliced lengthwise 1/2 inch thick

2-3 tablespoons water

2 medium red bell peppers, seeded and coarsely chopped

1 medium onion, coarsely chopped

1 cup chopped carrots

1/2 cup chopped celery

4 cloves garlic, chopped

8 ounces baby spinach

1 tablespoon Dr. Fuhrman's VegiZest or other no salt seasoning blend, adjusted to taste

2 cups no-salt-added or low sodium pasta sauce, divided

6 ounces nondairy mozzarella-type cheese, divided

DIRECTIONS

Preheat oven to 350° F. Lightly oil a non-stick baking pan. Arrange eggplant in a single layer in the pan. Bake about 20 minutes or until eggplant is flexible enough to roll up easily. Set aside.

Heat 2 tablespoons water in a large pan, add the bell pepper, onion, carrots, celery, and garlic; sauté until just tender, adding more water if needed. Add the spinach and VegiZest and cook until spinach is wilted.

Transfer to a mixing bowl. Mix in 2 to 3 tablespoons of the pasta sauce and all of the shredded cheese. Spread about 1/4 cup of the pasta sauce in a baking pan. Put some of the vegetable mixture on each eggplant slice, roll up and place in a pan. Pour the remaining sauce over the eggplant rolls. Bake for 20-30 minutes, until heated through.

PER SERVING: CALORIES 187; PROTEIN 9g; CARBOHYDRATES 32g; TOTAL FAT 4.3g; SATURATED FAT 1.2g; SODIUM 267mg; FIBER 10.2g; BETA-CAROTENE 4877ug; VITAMIN C 80mg; CALCIUM 259mg; IRON 2.6mg; FOLATE 153ug; MAGNESIUM 93mg; ZINC 1.5mg; SELENIUM 7.3ug

GARDEN STUFFED VEGETABLES

Serves: 6

INGREDIENTS

2 medium zucchini, cut in half lengthwise,
seeds and some meat removed, leaving shells intact

4 large peppers, assorted colors, tops sliced off, seeds removed

2 medium Portobello mushrooms, stems removed

1/2 cup quinoa, rinsed well

1 small red bell pepper, chopped

1/2 pound shiitake mushrooms, chopped

3 whole green onions, chopped

2 stalks celery, chopped

1 stalk broccoli, chopped in small pieces

4 cloves garlic, chopped in small pieces

1 cup cooked lentils* or canned, no-salt-added or low sodium, drained

1/2 cup coarsely chopped walnuts

2 ounces non-dairy mozzarella type cheese, shredded (see note)

1/2 cup raisins

1/4 cup plus 2 tablespoons chopped parsley, divided

2 teaspoons Bragg Liquid Aminos

1 tablespoon Dr. Fuhrman's MatoZest or other no salt seasoning blend, adjusted to taste

2 cups no-salt-added or low sodium pasta sauce

salad greens

1 tablespoon Dr. Fuhrman's Black Fig Vinegar or balsamic vinegar

DIRECTIONS

Preheat oven to 350° F.

On baking sheet, bake the zucchini and peppers for 5 minutes. Add portobello mushrooms and bake for an additional 15 minutes.

For filling:

Rinse the quinoa by placing it in a strainer and running water over it. Place the quinoa in a saucepot with one cup water. Bring to a boil, cover, reduce heat and let simmer for 13 to 15 minutes until all the water is absorbed. Set aside.

In small amount of water, sauté red pepper, shiitake mushrooms, green onions, celery, broccoli and garlic until vegetables are tender and water has cooked off.

In large bowl, mix cooked quinoa, lentils, walnuts, cheese substitute, raisins and 1/4 cup chopped parsley with sautéed ingredients and season with liquid aminos and MatoZest.

Fill zucchini, mushrooms and peppers with quinoa mixture and place in a baking dish.

Spoon pasta sauce over vegetables. Bake for 20-30 minutes until hot.

Serve on bed of salad greens which have been lightly tossed with Dr. Fuhrman's Black Fig vinegar or balsamic vinegar.

Garnish vegetables with remaining chopped parsley.

* Use 1/3 cup dry lentils. See cooking instructions on page 195.

Note: Daiya brand cheese substitute is a good choice.

PER SERVING: CALORIES 334; PROTEIN 15g; CARBOHYDRATES 53g; TOTAL FAT 9.7g; SATURATED FAT 1.3g; CHOLESTEROL 0.1mg; SODIUM 217mg; FIBER 11.8g; BETA-CAROTENE 2459ug; VITAMIN C 191mg; CALCIUM 193mg; IRON 5.8mg; FOLATE 269ug; MAGNESIUM 134mg; ZINC 3mg; SELENIUM 10.3ug

GARLICKY ZUCCHINI

Serves: 4

INGREDIENTS

6 cups sliced zucchini

3 cloves garlic, sliced

2 tablespoons water

1/4 teaspoon black pepper

1 tablespoon pine nuts

DIRECTIONS

Sauté zucchini and garlic in water over medium heat until tender, about 3 minutes. Add more water if necessary, to prevent scorching. Add black pepper and sprinkle with pine nuts.

PER SERVING: CALORIES 45; PROTEIN 3g; CARBOHYDRATES 7g; TOTAL FAT 1.8g; SATURATED FAT 0.2g; SODIUM 18mg; FIBER 2g; BETA-CAROTENE 204ug; VITAMIN C 30mg; CALCIUM 31mg; IRON 0.8mg; FOLATE 50ug; MAGNESIUM 35mg; ZINC 0.7mg; SELENIUM 0.7ug

GREAT GREENS

Serves: 4

INGREDIENTS

1 large bunch kale, tough stems and center ribs removed and leaves chopped

1 bunch Swiss chard, tough stems removed and leaves chopped

1 tablespoon Dr. Fuhrman's Spicy Pecan Vinegar or other flavored vinegar

1 clove garlic, minced

1/2 tablespoon Dr. Fuhrman's VegiZest or other no salt seasoning blend, adjusted to taste

1 teaspoon dried dill

1 teaspoon dried basil

black pepper to taste

DIRECTIONS

Steam the kale for 10 minutes. Add the Swiss chard and steam for another 10 minutes or until tender. Transfer to a bowl.

Combine the remaining ingredients and add to the greens. If desired, add 2 to 3 tablespoons of the steaming water to adjust consistency.

PER SERVING: CALORIES 46; PROTEIN 3g; CARBOHYDRATES 9g; TOTAL FAT 0.5g; SATURATED FAT 0.1g; SODIUM 150mg; FIBER 2.2g; BETA-CAROTENE 7435ug; VITAMIN C 86mg; CALCIUM 117mg; IRON 2.3mg; FOLATE 25ug; MAGNESIUM 68mg; ZINC 0.5mg; SELENIUM 1.1ug

GREEN MACHINE

Serves: 4

INGREDIENTS

2 large tomatoes, chopped

4 cloves garlic, chopped

1 medium onion, chopped

2 cups chopped shiitake mushrooms

1 bunch kale, tough stems removed, chopped

4 cups chopped bok choy

4 cups chopped broccoli rabe

DIRECTIONS

Add tomatoes, garlic, onions, and mushrooms to pan. Cover and simmer on low heat for 5 minutes. Add greens on top and continue to cook in covered pan on low heat for 10 more minutes or until vegetables are tender.

PER SERVING: CALORIES 106; PROTEIN 9g; CARBOHYDRATES 20g; TOTAL FAT 1.3g; SATURATED FAT 0.2g; SODIUM 74mg; FIBER 4.9g; BETA-CAROTENE 11273ug; VITAMIN C 165mg; CALCIUM 214mg; IRON 2.9mg; FOLATE 77ug; MAGNESIUM 63mg; ZINC 1.1mg; SELENIUM 6.5ug

HERBED BARLEY AND LENTILS

Serves: 4

INGREDIENTS

1/2 cup chopped onions

2 cloves garlic, chopped

1 cup hulled barley*

1/4 cup lentils

3 cups water

1/2 teaspoon Italian seasoning

1 tablespoon finely chopped fresh chives (or 1 teaspoon dried)

2 tablespoons finely chopped fresh basil (or 1/2 teaspoon dried)

DIRECTIONS

In a large saucepan, water sauté onions and garlic in a small amount of water until soft. Add remaining ingredients and bring to a boil. Reduce heat, cover and simmer for 1 hour or until barley and lentils are tender and water is absorbed.

Hulled barley is barley that has been minimally processed to remove only the tough inedible outer hull. Pearled barley receives additional processing and has a lower nutritional value.

PER SERVING: CALORIES 216; PROTEIN 9g; CARBOHYDRATES 43g; TOTAL FAT 1.2g; SATURATED FAT 0.3g; SODIUM 13mg; FIBER 12.1g; BETA-CAROTENE 70ug; VITAMIN C 3mg; CALCIUM 37mg; IRON 2.7mg; FOLATE 72ug; MAGNESIUM 81mg; ZINC 1.9mg; SELENIUM 18.7ug

ITALIAN STUFFER

Serves: 2

INGREDIENTS

2 cups shredded lettuce

1/4 cup chopped parsley

1/4 cup chopped unsalted, unsulfured dried tomatoes, soaked until soft

1/2 cup finely ground walnuts

1 teaspoon no-salt-added Italian seasoning

1 1/2 tablespoons tomato paste

pinch garlic powder

2 (100% whole grain) pitas or wraps

DIRECTIONS

In a bowl, combine lettuce, parsley, dried tomatoes, walnuts, Italian seasoning, tomato paste and garlic powder. Serve stuffed into a whole grain pita or wrap.

One to two ounces of oven baked white meat chicken or turkey, sliced or chopped may be added to each serving.

PER SERVING: CALORIES 363; PROTEIN 14g; CARBOHYDRATES 41g; TOTAL FAT 20.6g; SATURATED FAT 1.9g; SODIUM 558mg; FIBER 10g; BETA-CAROTENE 2511ug; VITAMIN C 30mg; CALCIUM 141mg; IRON 4.2mg; FOLATE 124ug; MAGNESIUM 117mg; ZINC 2.2mg; SELENIUM 2.7ug

KALE PESTO OVER PASTA AND BEANS

Serves: 6

INGREDIENTS

6 ounces whole wheat or brown rice penne pasta, cooked al dente

1 bunch kale, tough stems removed and chopped

1/2 cup pine nuts, lightly toasted*

5 cloves garlic, minced

1/4 cup unsweetened soy, hemp or almond milk

1 tablespoon fresh lemon juice

1 tablespoon olive oil

1/4 teaspoon crushed red pepper flakes

6 cups baby spinach

3 cups cooked cannellini beans* or 2 (15 ounce) cans cannellini beans low sodium or no-salt-added, drained

DIRECTIONS

Cook pasta according to package directions.

Steam kale until tender and pat dry. In a food processor, combine steamed kale, pine nuts, garlic, soy milk and lemon juice until a thick pesto is formed.

In a non-stick skillet, heat olive oil and red pepper flakes for 1 minute over medium heat. Add spinach and heat for 3 minutes or until spinach is soft. Add pesto.

Mix pasta and beans. Pour sauce over top.

* *Use 1 cup dry beans. See cooking instructions on page 195.*

* *Lightly toast pine nuts in a pan over medium heat for 3 minutes, shaking pan frequently.*

PER SERVING: CALORIES 446; PROTEIN 22g; CARBOHYDRATES 67g; TOTAL FAT 11.7g; SATURATED FAT 1.2g; SODIUM 43mg; FIBER 12g; BETA-CAROTENE 6535ug; VITAMIN C 115mg; CALCIUM 274mg; IRON 8.4mg; FOLATE 261ug; MAGNESIUM 179mg; ZINC 3.5mg; SELENIUM 20.8ug

LEMON ZEST SPINACH

Serves: 4

INGREDIENTS

1 1/4 pounds fresh spinach

6 cloves garlic, minced

5 tablespoons pine nuts, lightly toasted*

3 teaspoons lemon juice

1/2 teaspoon lemon zest

DIRECTIONS

Steam spinach and garlic until spinach is just wilted.

Place in bowl and toss in remaining ingredients.

* Lightly toast pine nuts in a pan over medium heat for 3 minutes, shaking pan frequently.

PER SERVING: CALORIES 123; PROTEIN 6g; CARBOHYDRATES 8g; TOTAL FAT 9.1g; SATURATED FAT 0.8g; SODIUM 113mg; FIBER 3.7g; BETA-CAROTENE 7977ug; VITAMIN C 43mg; CALCIUM 151mg; IRON 4.5mg; FOLATE 279ug; MAGNESIUM 140mg; ZINC 1.5mg; SELENIUM 2.1ug

MUSHROOM STROGANOFF

Serves: 4

INGREDIENTS

- 1 medium onion, chopped
- 1 clove garlic, minced
- 1 pound mushrooms, thinly sliced
- 2 tablespoons fresh lemon Juice
- 1 tablespoon fresh tarragon, chopped or 1 teaspoon dried tarragon
- 1 tablespoon sweet paprika
- 1 cup no-salt-added or low sodium vegetable broth
- 2 tablespoons tahini or pureed unhulled sesame seeds

DIRECTIONS

In a nonstick skillet, water sauté onion and garlic until soft. Add mushrooms and continue cooking until mushrooms soften and lose their moisture. Add lemon juice, tarragon and paprika and mix well.

Blend vegetable broth and tahini. (Heating the broth makes blending easier.)

Pour over mushroom mixture and mix well. Simmer until mixture thickens slightly or until desired consistency.

Spoon mixture over a bed of steamed kale or spinach or serve over smashed steamed cauliflower, parsnips or baked potato.

PER SERVING: CALORIES 101; PROTEIN 7g; CARBOHYDRATES 11g; TOTAL FAT 5g; SATURATED FAT 0.8g; SODIUM 29mg; FIBER 2.7g; BETA-CAROTENE 436ug; VITAMIN C 10mg; CALCIUM 41mg; IRON 1.9mg; FOLATE 37ug; MAGNESIUM 28mg; ZINC 1.2mg; SELENIUM 11ug

MEDITERRANEAN BEAN AND KALE SAUTÉ

Serves: 4

INGREDIENTS

1/2 cup unsulphured, no salt or oil added, sun-dried tomatoes, soaked in hot water for 30 minutes

2 bunches kale, tough stems and center ribs removed, chopped

1 medium onion, finely chopped

1 cup shiitake mushrooms, coarsely chopped

3 cloves garlic, pressed

1 tablespoon Dr. Fuhrman's VegiZest, or other no salt seasoning blend, adjusted to taste

1 cup cooked beans, any type or canned beans, no-salt-added or low sodium, drained

1 1/2 tablespoons Dr. Fuhrman's Riesling Reserve Vinegar or other fruity vinegar

1 tablespoon Dijon mustard

red pepper flakes, to taste

1/2 cup no-salt-added or low sodium pasta sauce

1/4 cup pine nuts, almonds or any type raw chopped nuts

1/8 cup non-dairy parmesan cheese

DIRECTIONS

Drain sun-dried tomatoes, reserving soaking water. Chop.

Heat tomato soaking water in a large skillet and sauté the kale, tomatoes, onion, mushrooms and garlic over medium heat for 5 minutes, adding additional water as needed. Add VegiZest, cover and steam for 10 minutes.

Add the beans, vinegar, mustard and red pepper flakes and cook for 3 more minutes or until mushrooms are tender and liquid cooks out.

Toss with pasta sauce. Serve topped with chopped nuts and non-dairy parmesan cheese.

PER SERVING: CALORIES 221; PROTEIN 10g; CARBOHYDRATES 32g; TOTAL FAT 7.3g; SATURATED FAT 0.7g; SODIUM 304mg; FIBER 7g; BETA-CAROTENE 6939ug; VITAMIN C 96mg; CALCIUM 173mg; IRON 3.9mg; FOLATE 85ug; MAGNESIUM 95mg; ZINC 1.9mg; SELENIUM 8.7ug

NO-MEAT BALLS

Serves: 6

INGREDIENTS

1/2 cup diced onion

3 cloves garlic, roasted and mashed

1/4 cup diced celery

2 tablespoons minced fresh parsley

1/4 teaspoon dried sage

1 teaspoon dried basil

1 teaspoon dried oregano

11/2 cup cooked lentils,
or 1 (15 ounce) can lentils, no-salt-added or low sodium, drained and rinsed

1/4 cup cooked brown rice

2-3 tablespoons tomato paste

1 tablespoon arrowroot powder or whole wheat flour

2 tablespoons MatoZest or other no salt seasoning blend, adjusted to taste

2 tablespoons nutritional yeast

freshly ground black pepper to taste

2 tablespoons vital wheat gluten flour for a chewier consistency (optional)

DIRECTIONS

Preheat oven to 350° F. Water sauté onion and garlic for 5 minutes. Add the celery, parsley, sage, basil and oregano. Sauté for another 5 minutes, adding more water as needed to prevent sticking.

In a large bowl, combine the sautéed vegetables with the remaining ingredients and mix well. Mash lightly with a potato masher.

With wet hands, form 2 tablespoons of the lentil mixture into a smooth ball. Repeat. Place the balls on a very lightly oiled baking sheet and bake for 20 minutes.

Serve with your favorite no-salt-added or low sodium marinara sauce.

Makes 18 balls.

PER SERVING: CALORIES 149; PROTEIN 11g; CARBOHYDRATES 27g; TOTAL FAT 0.5g; SATURATED FAT 0.1g; SODIUM 451mg; FIBER 7.4g; BETA-CAROTENE 826ug; VITAMIN C 11mg; CALCIUM 41mg; IRON 3.8mg; FOLATE 231ug; MAGNESIUM 59mg; ZINC 1.4mg; SELENIUM 7.2ug

No Pasta Vegetable Lasagna

Serves: 8

INGREDIENTS

For the LASAGNA "NOODLES":

2 large eggplants, sliced lengthwise 1/4 inch thick

3 small zucchini, sliced lengthwise as thinly as possible

3 small yellow squash, sliced lengthwise as thinly as possible

For the TOFU RICOTTA:

16 ounces silken tofu

1 small onion, cut into quarters

4 cloves garlic, cut in half

1 cup fresh basil leaves

1 1/4 pounds firm tofu, squeezed dry and crumbled

1/4 cup Dr. Fuhrman's MatoZest, or other no-salt seasoning blend, adjusted to taste

2 tablespoons dried Italian herbs

1 cup grated nondairy mozzarella cheese*

For the VEGETABLES:

2 heads broccoli, coarsely chopped

4 cups sliced mixed fresh mushrooms (shiitake, cremini, oyster)

4 medium bell peppers (red, yellow and/or orange) seeded and chopped

7 ounces baby spinach

3 cups no-salt-added or low sodium pasta sauce, divided

shredded fresh basil for garnish

DIRECTIONS

To make the lasagna noodles, preheat the oven to 350° F. Wipe a baking pan with a small amount of olive oil. Place the eggplant, zucchini, and yellow squash in the pan and bake for 10 minutes, or until flexible but not completely cooked. Work in batches if necessary. Set aside.

While the "noodles" are baking, make the tofu "ricotta". Puree the silken tofu, onion, and garlic in a food processor or high-powered blender. Add the basil leaves and pulse to coarsely chop. Transfer to a medium bowl and mix in the crumbled firm tofu. Add the MatoZest, Italian seasoning, and grated nondairy cheese. Set aside.

To prepare the vegetables, sauté broccoli, mushrooms, bell peppers and spinach without water, over low heat for 5 minutes, just until tender.

To assemble the lasagna, spread a thin layer of the pasta sauce on the bottom of a baking dish. Layer the eggplant slices, sautéed vegetables, yellow squash slices, zucchini slices and tofu "ricotta" and then spread with pasta sauce. Repeat the layers, ending with the tofu "ricotta". Spread the remaining pasta sauce on top and bake at 350° F, uncovered, for 1 hour, or until hot and bubbly. Garnish with the shredded basil.

* Daiya brand is a good choice

PER SERVING: CALORIES 376; PROTEIN 18g; CARBOHYDRATES 63g; TOTAL FAT 9.8g; SATURATED FAT 1.6g; SODIUM 229mg; FIBER 15g; BETA-CAROTENE 3129ug; VITAMIN C 213mg; CALCIUM 367mg; IRON 6.1mg; FOLATE 248ug; MAGNESIUM 167mg; ZINC 2.8mg; SELENIUM 25.8ug

ORANGE SESAME KALE

Serves: 4

INGREDIENTS

1/2 cup raw cashew butter or 1 cup raw cashews

2/3 cup orange juice

2 teaspoons Dr. Fuhrman's VegiZest,
or other no-salt-added seasoning blend, adjusted to taste

2 bunches kale, leaves removed from tough stems and chopped

2 tablespoons unhulled sesame seeds, lightly toasted*

DIRECTIONS

Whisk together cashew butter, orange juice, and VegiZest or if using cashews, blend together in a high powered blender.

Steam kale for 15 to 20 minutes, stirring halfway through cooking.

Combine steamed kale and cashew mixture.

Sprinkle with toasted sesame seeds.

* *Lightly toast sesame seeds in a pan over medium heat, shaking pan frequently, about 2 minutes or until lightly browned.*

PER SERVING: CALORIES 343; PROTEIN 12g; CARBOHYDRATES 22g; TOTAL FAT 26.1g; SATURATED FAT 5g; SODIUM 46mg; FIBER 3.1g; BETA-CAROTENE 6740ug; VITAMIN C 86mg; CALCIUM 122mg; IRON 4mg; FOLATE 57ug; MAGNESIUM 162mg; ZINC 3.2mg; SELENIUM 6.2ug

PASTA WITH ROASTED VEGETABLES

Serves: 6

INGREDIENTS

2 red bell peppers, cut into 1/2 inch pieces

1 medium eggplant, unpeeled, cut into 1/2 inch pieces

1 large yellow crookneck squash, cut into 1/2 inch pieces

1 1/2 cups peeled butternut squash, cut into 1/2 inch pieces

2 tablespoons olive oil, divided

1 pound whole wheat or whole grain pasta

2 medium tomatoes, seeded, diced

1/2 cup chopped fresh basil or 1 1/2 tablespoons dried basil

2 tablespoons balsamic vinegar or 1 tablespoon fresh lemon juice

2 cloves garlic, minced

DIRECTIONS

Preheat oven to 450° F.

Wipe large roasting pan with a thin coating of olive oil. Combine red bell peppers, eggplant, yellow squash, and butternut squash in prepared pan. Drizzle with 1 tablespoon olive oil and toss to coat.

Roast until vegetables are tender and beginning to brown, stirring occasionally, about 25 minutes.

Meanwhile, cook pasta and drain, reserving 1/2 cup cooking liquid.

Combine pasta, roasted vegetables, tomatoes, and basil in large bowl.

Add remaining tablespoon of oil, vinegar and garlic. Toss to combine.

Add cooking liquid by tablespoons to moisten, if desired.

PER SERVING: CALORIES 365; PROTEIN 14g; CARBOHYDRATES 71g; TOTAL FAT 6g; SATURATED FAT 0.9g; SODIUM 14mg; FIBER 5.7g; BETA-CAROTENE 2450ug; VITAMIN C 69mg; CALCIUM 74mg; IRON 3.7mg; FOLATE 104ug; MAGNESIUM 149mg; ZINC 2.3mg; SELENIUM 55.9ug

PORTOBELLO RED PEPPER SANDWICH

Serves: 4 — Prep Time: 25 minutes

INGREDIENTS

SANDWICH:

> 1/2 large red onion, thinly sliced
>
> 4 large Portobello mushrooms, stems removed
>
> 4 (100% whole grain) pitas
>
> 2 cups large arugula leaves
>
> 2 medium drained, roasted red bell peppers, from jar, seeded and cut into 1/2-inch-thick slices

TAHINI SPREAD:

> 1/2 cup tahini (pureed sesame seeds) or 2/3 cup unhulled sesame seeds
>
> 1/2 cup water
>
> 1 tablespoon fresh lemon juice
>
> 1 tablespoon Dr. Fuhrman's VegiZest or other no salt seasoning blend, adjusted to taste
>
> 1 teaspoon Bragg Liquid Aminos or low sodium soy sauce
>
> 2 dates, pitted and chopped
>
> 1 small clove garlic, chopped

DIRECTIONS

Preheat oven to 375° F. Arrange mushrooms and onions on baking sheet and roast until tender, about 15 to 20 minutes.

Meanwhile, make tahini spread by blending all ingredients together until creamy in a food processor or high powered blender. (If using whole sesame seeds, blend sesame seeds with 1/4 cup of water until creamy and then add the other 1/4 cup water and remaining ingredients).

Split pitas in half horizontally and warm slightly. Spread generous amount of tahini spread on top half of split pita. Place 1/2 cup arugula on bottom half and then 1 mushroom cap (pat dry with paper towels to absorb liquid), sliced onion and roasted red pepper.

PER SERVING: CALORIES 392; PROTEIN 14g; CARBOHYDRATES 52g; TOTAL FAT 18g; SATURATED FAT 2.5g; SODIUM 442mg; FIBER 7.7g; BETA-CAROTENE 443ug; VITAMIN C 7mg; CALCIUM 80mg; IRON 4mg; FOLATE 78ug; MAGNESIUM 87mg; ZINC 2.8mg; SELENIUM 35.2ug

PORTOBELLO WRAPS WITH WATERCRESS SALSA

Serves: 2

INGREDIENTS

4 Portobello mushroom caps, cut into strips

1 bunch watercress, tough stems removed, chopped

1/4 cup chopped red onion

1 clove garlic, minced

1 tablespoon Dr. Fuhrman's Black Fig Vinegar or balsamic vinegar

1 tablespoon fresh lime juice

1 ripe avocado, peeled, pitted and diced

4 cups chopped romaine lettuce or mixed baby greens

2 large (100% whole grain) tortillas

DIRECTIONS

Heat 2 tablespoons water in a skillet and water sauté mushrooms until tender, about 5 minutes.

Meanwhile, combine watercress, onion, garlic, vinegar and lime juice. Fold in avocado.

Top each tortilla with lettuce, cooked mushrooms and watercress mixture.

Roll up.

PER SERVING: CALORIES 320; PROTEIN 10g; CARBOHYDRATES 39g; TOTAL FAT 16.2g; SATURATED FAT 2.5g; SODIUM 245mg; FIBER 11.8g; BETA-CAROTENE 4917ug; VITAMIN C 53mg; CALCIUM 152mg; IRON 3.7mg; FOLATE 300ug; MAGNESIUM 74mg; ZINC 2mg; SELENIUM 24.1ug

Pistachio Crusted Tempeh with Balsamic Glazed Shiitakes

Serves: 4

INGREDIENTS

8 ounces tempeh, diagonally sliced, as thinly as possible

1 pound shiitake mushrooms, stemmed, thinly sliced

MARINADE:

2 cloves garlic, minced

1 tablespoon chopped fresh basil

1 tablespoon chopped fresh cilantro

pinch hot pepper flakes

1 cup no-salt-added or low sodium vegetable broth

2 tablespoons balsamic vinegar

1 teaspoon Bragg Liquid Aminios or low sodium soy sauce

CRUST:

1 cup pistachios, shelled

4 tablespoons corn meal

2 tablespoons nutritional yeast

1 teaspoon onion powder

1 teaspoon garlic powder

DIRECTIONS

Place tempeh in a saucepan with water to cover, simmer for 10 minutes.

Combine ingredients for marinade. Remove tempeh from water and add to marinade. Marinate for at least one hour.

Preheat oven to 400° F. Process pistachios in food processor until finely chopped. Add remaining crust ingredients and pulse until thoroughly mixed. Place in large shallow bowl. Remove tempeh from marinade and drain. Reserve marinade. Dip in tempeh in crust mixture to coat.

Place crusted tempeh and sliced mushrooms side by side on a rimmed baking sheet. Spoon 2-3 tablespoons of marinade over mushrooms. Bake for 13 minutes or until mushrooms are soft, turning occasionally.

Simmer remaining marinade for 2 minutes. Drizzle tempeh and mushrooms with marinade before serving.

PER SERVING: CALORIES 374; PROTEIN 24g; CARBOHYDRATES 30g; TOTAL FAT 20.7g; SATURATED FAT 3.1g; SODIUM 98mg; FIBER 6.1g; BETA-CAROTENE 173ug; VITAMIN C 5mg; CALCIUM 120mg; IRON 4.7mg; FOLATE 225ug; MAGNESIUM 109mg; ZINC 2.4mg; SELENIUM 14.2ug

PITA STUFFED WITH SEASONED GREENS

Serves: 1

INGREDIENTS

5-6 large leaves kale, Swiss chard or mustard greens, tough stems removed

1 teaspoon lemon juice

1 (100% whole grain) pita

dash garlic powder

2 thin slices red onion

sliced tomato

low sodium mustard, as desired

DIRECTIONS

Steam the greens until tender, about 10-15 minutes. Sprinkle with lemon juice and garlic powder.

Stuff whole grain pita with greens, red onion and tomato. Add mustard if desired.

Note: Sandwich can also be topped with Russian Fig Dressing: Blend 3 tablespoons no-salt-added or low sodium pasta sauce, 1 tablespoon raw almond butter and 1 tablespoon Dr.Fuhrman's Black Fig Vinegar.

PER SERVING: CALORIES 194; PROTEIN 8g; CARBOHYDRATES 40g; TOTAL FAT 1.8g; SATURATED FAT 0.3g; SODIUM 544mg; FIBER 7.1g; BETA-CAROTENE 4141ug; VITAMIN C 23mg; CALCIUM 76mg; IRON 4.5mg; FOLATE 33ug; MAGNESIUM 142mg; ZINC 1.4mg; SELENIUM 29.2ug

QUICK VEGETABLE BEAN MEDLEY

Serves: 4

INGREDIENTS

1 head broccoli, small florets, with peeled and sliced 1/2" thick stems

1 red bell pepper, thinly sliced

8 cloves garlic, chopped

1/2 pound shiitake mushrooms, sliced

3 cups cooked red beans* or 2 (15 ounce) cans,
no-salt-added or low sodium, drained

1 tablespoon Dr. Fuhrman's VegiZest,
or other no salt seasoning blend, adjusted to taste

1/2 cup raw sunflower seeds, lightly toasted

DIRECTIONS

In large pan, heat 1/8 cup water, add broccoli, red pepper, garlic and mushrooms, cover and sauté vegetables until tender, about 10 minutes. Add beans and VegiZest and continue cooking, uncovered for an additional 5 minutes, adding more water if necessary. Top with sunflower seeds.

* Use 1 cup dry beans. See cooking instructions on page 195.

PER SERVING: CALORIES 413; PROTEIN 28g; CARBOHYDRATES 65g; TOTAL FAT 8.2g; SATURATED FAT 0.9g; SODIUM 56mg; FIBER 16.2g; BETA-CAROTENE 783ug; VITAMIN C 177mg; CALCIUM 164mg; IRON 7.4mg; FOLATE 427ug; MAGNESIUM 149mg; ZINC 3.7mg; SELENIUM 12.8ug

ROASTED VEGETABLE PIZZA

Serves: 2

INGREDIENTS

2 cups broccoli florets

1 large red bell pepper, sliced 1 inch thick

1 large Portobello mushroom, cut into 1/2 inch slices

1 teaspoon garlic powder

1 tablespoon balsamic vinegar

1 teaspoon Mrs. Dash seasoning or Spike no salt seasoning

5 ounces baby spinach

2 (100% whole grain) tortillas or pitas

1/2 cup no-salt-added or low sodium pasta sauce

2 ounces mozzarella type non-dairy cheese, shredded

DIRECTIONS

Preheat oven to 350° F.

Toss broccoli, bell peppers, and mushrooms with garlic powder, balsamic vinegar, and seasoning. Roast seasoned vegetables on a cookie sheet for 30 minutes, turning occasionally and mounding to keep from drying out.

Steam spinach until just wilted.

Remove vegetables when done and preheat oven to 400° F.

Spread a thin layer of pasta sauce on tortilla, sprinkle non-dairy cheese, and distribute roasted vegetables and spinach on top.

Bake for approximately 7 minutes or until cheese is melted and tortilla is lightly brown around edges.

PER SERVING: CALORIES 396; PROTEIN 17g; CARBOHYDRATES 64g; TOTAL FAT 9.5g; SATURATED FAT 2.5g; SODIUM 632mg; FIBER 6.6g; BETA-CAROTENE 5281ug; VITAMIN C 172mg; CALCIUM 321mg; IRON 6.1mg; FOLATE 318ug; MAGNESIUM 127mg; ZINC 2.2mg; SELENIUM 29.4ug

SPAGHETTI SQUASH PRIMAVERA

Serves: 4

INGREDIENTS

1 medium spaghetti squash

1 1/2 carrots, diagonally sliced

1/2 cup diagonally sliced celery

3 cloves garlic, minced

1 1/2 cups shredded cabbage

1 small zucchini, chopped into small pieces

1 1/2 cups cooked pinto beans*,
or 1 (15 ounce) can pinto beans, no-salt-added or low sodium, drained

1 1/2 cups chopped tomatoes
or 1 (15 ounce) can no-salt-added or low sodium, drained

1/3 cup no-salt-added or low sodium vegetable broth

1 teaspoon dried thyme

1 teaspoon dried parsley

1 cup no-salt-added or low sodium pasta sauce

1 head romaine lettuce leaves

DIRECTIONS

Preheat oven to 350° F. Slice spaghetti squash in half lengthwise; remove seeds. Place both halves upside down on a baking sheet. Bake for 45 minutes or until tender.

Meanwhile, cook carrots and celery in 2 tablespoons of water in a covered pan over medium heat for 10 minutes, stirring occasionally. Add a little more water if needed. Add garlic, cabbage, and zucchini and cook, covered, for another 10 minutes. Stir in remaining ingredients, except for pasta sauce. Cover and simmer for 10 minutes or until carrots are tender.

When squash is done, remove from oven and using a fork, scrape spaghetti-like strands from squash into a bowl. Add pasta sauce and combine by mixing thoroughly. Mix the vegetables, beans and herbs with the squash/ pasta sauce mixture and serve on a bed of shredded romaine lettuce, if desired, or place back in the hollowed out squash bowls.

*Use 1/2 cup dried beans. See bean cooking instructions on page 195.

PER SERVING: CALORIES 268; PROTEIN 13g; CARBOHYDRATES 51g; TOTAL FAT 4.5g; SATURATED FAT 0.7g; SODIUM 94mg; FIBER 14.6g; BETA-CAROTENE 5555ug; VITAMIN C 63mg; CALCIUM 158mg; IRON 4.3mg; FOLATE 291ug; MAGNESIUM 101mg; ZINC 1.7mg; SELENIUM 6.1ug

SPEEDY VEGETABLE WRAP

Serves: 2

INGREDIENTS

2 (100% whole grain) tortillas or pitas

1 tablespoon fat free, low sodium dressing

2 cups broccoli slaw mix

1 large tomato, diced

2 tablespoons shredded non-dairy cheese

DIRECTIONS

Spread dressing over tortillas. Add broccoli slaw mix, tomatoes, and non-dairy cheese.

Place in toaster oven or microwave just long enough to melt the cheese. Roll up tortillas enclosing filling.

If making pitas, stuff with dressing, vegetable, and cheese and serve without heating.

Note: Prepackaged broccoli slaw can be purchased in the produce section of many markets. Cole slaw mix, shredded cabbage, or shredded broccoli may also be used.

PER SERVING: CALORIES 263; PROTEIN 14g; CARBOHYDRATES 47g; TOTAL FAT 4.5g; SATURATED FAT 0.7g; CHOLESTEROL 0.2mg; SODIUM 497mg; FIBER 7.9g; BETA-CAROTENE 2814ug; VITAMIN C 68mg; CALCIUM 113mg; IRON 4.3mg; FOLATE 85ug; MAGNESIUM 133mg; ZINC 1.9mg; SELENIUM 34.6ug

Spinach and Brussels Sprouts Delight

Serves: 4

INGREDIENTS

1 pound Brussels sprouts, cut in half

14 ounces baby spinach

4 cloves garlic, minced

1 small onion, chopped

1 1/2 cups chopped tomatoes
or 1 (15 ounce) can no-salt-added or low sodium chopped tomatoes

1 tablespoon Dr. Fuhrman's VegiZest or other no salt seasoning blend,
adjusted to taste

DIRECTIONS

Steam Brussels sprouts for 8 minutes. Add spinach and continue to
steam until spinach is wilted and the Brussels sprouts are almost tender.
Meanwhile, heat 2 tablespoons water in a large pot and water sauté the
garlic and onion until the onion is tender, about 5 minutes. Add the Brussels
sprouts and spinach, chopped tomatoes and VegiZest. Simmer for 10
minutes.

PER SERVING: CALORIES 110; PROTEIN 11g; CARBOHYDRATES 22g; TOTAL FAT 1g; SATURATED FAT 0.2g;
SODIUM 124mg; FIBER 8.2g; BETA-CAROTENE 6838ug; VITAMIN C 141mg; CALCIUM 168mg; IRON 4.8mg;
FOLATE 282ug; MAGNESIUM 119mg; ZINC 1.3mg; SELENIUM 3.4ug

SPINACH STUFFED MUSHROOMS

Serves: 3

INGREDIENTS

1 small onion, chopped

12 large mushrooms, stems removed and chopped

1 clove garlic, minced

1/2 teaspoon dried thyme

1/4 cup no-salt-added or low sodium vegetable broth

5 ounces fresh spinach

2 tablespoons raw almond butter

1 tablespoon nutritional yeast

1/4 teaspoon black pepper, or to taste

DIRECTIONS

Preheat oven to 350° F.

In a large pan, heat 2-3 tablespoons of water and water sauté chopped onion for 2 minutes, add mushroom stems, garlic and thyme and continue to sauté until onions and mushrooms are tender, about 3 minutes. Add mushroom caps to pan, along with vegetable broth, bring to a simmer and cook for 5 minutes.

Remove mushroom caps from pan and place on a lightly oiled baking sheet. Add spinach to onion mixture remaining in pan and heat until wilted. Remove from heat and stir in almond butter, nutritional yeast and black pepper.

Fill mushroom caps with spinach/onion mixture and bake for 15-20 minutes or until golden brown.

PER SERVING: CALORIES 121; PROTEIN 7g; CARBOHYDRATES 12g; TOTAL FAT 6.8g; SATURATED FAT 0.7g; SODIUM 53mg; FIBER 3.8g; BETA-CAROTENE 2664ug; VITAMIN C 18mg; CALCIUM 99mg; IRON 3mg; FOLATE 222ug; MAGNESIUM 86mg; ZINC 1.3mg; SELENIUM 7.5ug

STEAMED ARTICHOKES

Serves: 2

INGREDIENTS

4 artichokes

DIRECTIONS

Select heavy artichokes that squeak slightly when squeezed. Slice one inch off the top of each artichoke. Cut off the very bottom of the stem, but keep the stem attached. Slice artichokes in half lengthwise. Place them in a steamer basket over several inches of water. Bring water to boil, cover and steam for 40 minutes. Set aside until cool enough to handle.

Scoop out and discard the fibrous choke from the center of the artichoke. Eat heart as well as the tender insides of each leaf.

PER SERVING: CALORIES 120; PROTEIN 8g; CARBOHYDRATES 27g; TOTAL FAT 0.4g; SATURATED FAT 0.1g; SODIUM 241mg; FIBER 13.8g; BETA-CAROTENE 271ug; VITAMIN C 30mg; CALCIUM 113mg; IRON 3.3mg; FOLATE 174ug; MAGNESIUM 154mg; ZINC 1.3mg; SELENIUM 0.5ug

SWISS CHARD AND SWEET POTATO GRATIN

Serves: 6

INGREDIENTS

1 teaspoon chopped fresh ginger

1 small onion, finely chopped

1/2 cup chopped green bell pepper

8 cups Swiss chard, stems removed, coarsely chopped

4 medium (about 1 1/4 pounds) sweet potatoes, peeled, sliced 1/8 inch thick

8 ounces tempeh, sliced as thinly as possible

2 cups unsweetened hemp, soy or almond milk

1/8 teaspoon nutmeg

1/8 teaspoon black pepper

1/4 cup non-dairy mozzarella-type cheese

2 tablespoons flax seeds, toasted

DIRECTIONS

Preheat oven to 400° F. Rub 9 X 13 baking dish with a small amount of olive oil.

Heat 1/8 cup water in a large pan and water sauté ginger, onion, and green pepper until softened. Add Swiss chard and cook until just tender.

Arrange one third sliced sweet potatoes on bottom of prepared baking dish. Place one half of tempeh and one half of Swiss chard mixture on top. Arrange another one third sweet potato slices and remaining tempeh and Swiss chard, followed by remaining sweet potato.

Combine milk, nutmeg and black pepper. Pour over dish. Cover with foil and bake for 35 minutes. Remove foil, top with non-dairy cheese and bake for an additional 15 minutes. Sprinkle with toasted flax seeds.

PER SERVING: CALORIES 349; PROTEIN 21g; CARBOHYDRATES 46g; TOTAL FAT 11.1g; SATURATED FAT 2g; SODIUM 347mg; FIBER 8.4g; BETA-CAROTENE 14167ug; VITAMIN C 42mg; CALCIUM 245mg; IRON 5.3mg; FOLATE 68ug; MAGNESIUM 188mg; ZINC 2.2mg; SELENIUM 9.6ug

Swiss Chard with Garlic and Lemon

Serves: 4

INGREDIENTS

2 pounds Swiss chard, tough stems and center ribs removed, chopped

1/8 cup water

3 cloves garlic, chopped

1 tablespoon lemon juice

1/4 teaspoon ground pepper

DIRECTIONS

In a large pan, sauté Swiss chard in water over medium heat until slightly wilted, about 1 minute, adding more water as necessary to prevent scorching. Stir in garlic. Cover and cook until tender, about 3 minutes, stirring occasionally. Uncover and cook another 1-2 minutes until liquid evaporates. Stir in lemon juice and pepper.

PER SERVING: CALORIES 37; PROTEIN 3g; CARBOHYDRATES 8g; TOTAL FAT 0.4g; SATURATED FAT 0.1g; SODIUM 363mg; FIBER 2.8g; BETA-CAROTENE 6204ug; VITAMIN C 54mg; CALCIUM 92mg; IRON 3.1mg; FOLATE 24ug; MAGNESIUM 139mg; ZINC 0.6mg; SELENIUM 1.9ug

SUPREME KALE

Serves: 4

INGREDIENTS

1 small onion, thinly sliced

1 clove garlic, chopped

1/4 teaspoon crushed red pepper flakes

1 bunch kale, leaves removed from tough stems and chopped

2 carrots, shredded or sliced thin with a vegetable peeler

1 tablespoon toasted sesame seeds

DIRECTIONS

In a large pan, water sauté onion, garlic and red pepper flakes for 1 minute. Add half of kale, stir for 1 minute then add remaining kale and cook until softened. Use a small amount of water as needed to prevent sticking. Add shredded carrots and continue cooking 2-4 minutes until kale is tender.

Toss with sesame seeds.

PER SERVING: CALORIES 110; PROTEIN 4g; CARBOHYDRATES 20g; TOTAL FAT 2.6g; SATURATED FAT 0.4g; SODIUM 77mg; FIBER 5g; BETA-CAROTENE 11595ug; VITAMIN C 93mg; CALCIUM 136mg; IRON 1.8mg; FOLATE 46ug; MAGNESIUM 51mg; ZINC 1mg; SELENIUM 1.3ug

Sweet Potato Fries

Serves: 4

INGREDIENTS

4 sweet potatoes

1 tablespoon garlic powder

1 tablespoon onion powder

DIRECTIONS

Preheat oven to 400° F. Peel sweet potatoes if not organic. Cut into strips. Lay on a non-stick cookie sheet. Sprinkle garlic powder and onion powder on potatoes. Bake approximately 45 minutes, turning potatoes every 15 minutes or until tender and lightly browned.

PER SERVING: CALORIES 124; PROTEIN 3g; CARBOHYDRATES 29g; TOTAL FAT 0.1g; SODIUM 73mg; FIBER 4.2g; BETA-CAROTENE 11062ug; VITAMIN C 4mg; CALCIUM 46mg; IRON 0.9mg; FOLATE 17ug; MAGNESIUM 36mg; ZINC 0.5mg; SELENIUM 1.6ug

THAI VEGETABLE CURRY

Serves: 6

INGREDIENTS

4 cloves garlic, finely chopped

2 tablespoons finely chopped fresh ginger

2 tablespoons chopped fresh mint

2 tablespoons chopped fresh basil

2 tablespoons chopped fresh cilantro

2 cups carrot juice, fresh (2 pounds of carrots, juiced) or bottled

1 red bell pepper, seeded and thinly sliced

1 large eggplant, peeled, if desired & cut into 1 inch cubes

2 cups green beans, cut in 2 inch pieces

3 cups sliced shiitake mushrooms

1 (8 ounce) can bamboo shoots, drained

2 tablespoons Dr. Fuhrman's VegiZest
or other no salt seasoning blend, adjusted to taste

1/2 teaspoon curry powder

2 cups watercress leaves, divided

3 tablespoons unsalted natural chunky peanut butter

2 pounds firm tofu, cut into 1/4 inch thick slices

1/2 cup unsweetened light coconut milk

1/4 cup slivered raw almonds

mint, basil or cilantro leaves, for garnish

DIRECTIONS

Place the garlic, ginger, mint, basil, cilantro, carrot juice, bell pepper, eggplant, green beans, mushrooms, bamboo shoots, VegiZest, curry powder, and 1 cup of the watercress in a wok or large skillet. Bring to a boil, cover and simmer, stirring occasionally, until all the vegetables are tender.

Mix in the peanut butter. Add the tofu, bring to a simmer, and toss until hot. Add the coconut milk and heat through.

Top with the remaining 1 cup watercress and the almonds. Garnish with mint, basil or cilantro leaves, if desired.

Note: This can be served over brown rice or quinoa. Frozen vegetables may be used instead of fresh.

PER SERVING: CALORIES 375; PROTEIN 15g; CARBOHYDRATES 48g; TOTAL FAT 16.9g; SATURATED FAT 6.1g; SODIUM 108mg; FIBER 8.6g; BETA-CAROTENE 8642ug; VITAMIN C 51mg; CALCIUM 205mg; IRON 5.3mg; FOLATE 114ug; MAGNESIUM 138mg; ZINC 3mg; SELENIUM 26.3ug

THANKSGIVING NON-MEAT LOAF

Serves: 6

INGREDIENTS

2 tablespoons arrowroot powder

4 tablespoons water

2 teaspoons Bragg Liquid Aminos

1 box soft tofu, drained and patted dry with paper towel

3/4 cup chopped walnuts

1 1/4 cups chopped onions

1/2 cup chopped celery

2 cups chopped Portobello mushrooms

1 tablespoon water

1 tablespoon Dr. Fuhrman's VegiZest,
or other no-salt seasoning blend, adjusted to taste

2 teaspoons Spike (no salt)

1 1/2 teaspoons oregano

1 1/2 teaspoons basil

1/2 teaspoon sage

3/4 cup whole grain bread crumbs

1 1/2 cups cooked brown rice

DIRECTIONS

Preheat oven to 350° F.

Mix arrowroot powder, water, Bragg liquid aminos, and tofu together in a high-powered blender. Add walnuts & blend until smooth.

Sauté onions, celery, and mushrooms in water with seasonings and herbs until vegetables are soft, stirring occasionally. In a bowl, mix together tofu mixture, vegetables, bread crumbs and cooked rice.

With a paper towel, spread a small amount of olive oil in a loaf pan. Add mixture to pan and bake for 1 hour and 15 minutes. Let cool for 30 minutes. Turn loaf out and slice.

Note: May be served with low sodium ketchup.

PER SERVING: CALORIES 350; PROTEIN 15g; CARBOHYDRATES 47g; TOTAL FAT 13.3g; SATURATED FAT 1.5g; CHOLESTEROL 0.2mg; SODIUM 359mg; FIBER 5.3g; BETA-CAROTENE 70ug; VITAMIN C 4mg; CALCIUM 143mg; IRON 3.1mg; FOLATE 107ug; MAGNESIUM 96mg; ZINC 3mg; SELENIUM 14.2ug

VEGETABLE BEAN BURRITO

Serves: 6

INGREDIENTS

1 head broccoli florets, chopped

1/2 head cauliflower florets, chopped

2 carrots, chopped

2 medium red bell peppers, seeded and chopped

1 medium zucchini, chopped

1 medium onion, chopped

4 cloves garlic, chopped

1 1/2 tablespoons Dr. Fuhrman's VegiZest,
or other no salt seasoning blend, adjusted to taste

1 teaspoon dried basil

1 teaspoon dried oregano

1 teaspoon dried parsley

1/2 cup raw cashews

1/2 cup raw almonds

1/2 cup unsweetened soy, hemp or almond milk

1 1/2 cups cooked pinto beans
or 1 (15 ounce) can pinto beans, no-salt-added or low sodium, drained

6 (100% whole grain) tortillas or large romaine lettuce leaves

low sodium or no-salt-added salsa

DIRECTIONS

Place 2 tablespoons water, the broccoli, cauliflower, carrot, bell pepper, zucchini, onion, garlic, VegiZest, basil, oregano, and parsley in a large covered pot. Sauté for 15 minutes or until tender, adding more water if needed. In the meantime, place nuts and milk in a food processor or high-powered blender and blend until smooth. Add the cashew mixture and beans to the vegetables and mix thoroughly. Spread the mixture on the tortillas and roll up to form burritos. Serve with salsa.

PER SERVING: CALORIES 524; PROTEIN 20g; CARBOHYDRATES 78g; TOTAL FAT 17.2g; SATURATED FAT 3.6g; SODIUM 447mg; FIBER 14.7g; BETA-CAROTENE 3666ug; VITAMIN C 167mg; CALCIUM 154mg; IRON 6.2mg; FOLATE 385ug; MAGNESIUM 151mg; ZINC 3.2mg; SELENIUM 25.8ug

VEGETABLE GARBANZO WRAPS

Serves: 4

INGREDIENTS

1 large tomato, chopped

1 avocado, chopped

1 cucumber, chopped

4 leaves romaine lettuce, shredded

1 1/2 cups garbanzo beans*, mashed
or 1 (15 ounce) can garbanzo beans no-salt-added
or low sodium, drained and mashed

2 tablespoons Dr. Fuhrman's Riesling Reserve Vinegar
or other fruit flavored vinegar

4 (100% whole grain) tortillas

1/2 tablespoon raw sesame tahini

DIRECTIONS

Toss vegetables with garbanzo beans and vinegar.

Warm a whole grain tortilla, spread a thin coating of tahini on it, and roll with the vegetable/bean mixture.

* Use 1/3 cup dry beans. See cooking instructions on page 195.

PER SERVING: CALORIES 473; PROTEIN 17g; CARBOHYDRATES 71g; TOTAL FAT 15.6g; SATURATED FAT 3.1g; SODIUM 361mg; FIBER 13.6g; BETA-CAROTENE 2237ug; VITAMIN C 35mg; CALCIUM 111mg; IRON 5.3mg; FOLATE 311ug; MAGNESIUM 92mg; ZINC 2.2mg; SELENIUM 19.6ug

VEGETABLE SHEPHERD'S PIE

Serves: 6

INGREDIENTS

4 large sweet potatoes

1 cup fresh or frozen chopped broccoli

1 cup fresh or frozen sliced cauliflower

1 medium chopped leek

1 red bell pepper, cut into 1" squares

1 teaspoon herb de Provence (dried French herbs)

4 tablespoons Dr. Fuhrman's VegiZest,
or other no salt seasoning blend, such as Mrs.Dash, adjusted to taste

2 cups fresh chopped spinach or 1 cup frozen, thawed and drained

1/2 cup carrot juice

4 teaspoons cornstarch

1 cup firm tofu, water squeezed out and crumbled

1 cup finely chopped hazelnuts, brazil nuts, or raw almonds

2 tablespoons chopped fresh parsley, for garnish

DIRECTIONS

Preheat oven to 375° F. Bake sweet potatoes until soft, about 45 minutes. When potatoes are tender, peel and mash. Set aside.

Place broccoli, cauliflower, leeks, bell peppers, herb de Provence, and Dr. Fuhrman's VegiZest in a large sauté pan along with 2 cups of water. Simmer until almost tender, about 10 minutes. (If using frozen broccoli and cauliflower, reduce water to 1 1/2 cups) Add fresh or thawed, drained frozen spinach and toss.

Drain and remove vegetables, reserving vegetable liquid in pot. Whisk cornstarch into carrot juice and whisk into boiling vegetable liquid until it thickens. Add vegetables and crumbled tofu to sauce and toss to combine.

Divide mixture into two 8-inch pie pans. Top each with 1/4 cup nuts. Spread sweet potatoes over the top and sprinkle with remaining nuts.

Bake at 375° F for 20-30 minutes until hot and nuts are lightly browned. If desired, sprinkle with parsley.

This dish may be prepared ahead and frozen, unbaked. Cover tightly with aluminum foil before freezing. Do not defrost, but bake an additional 10 to 15 minutes.

PER SERVING: CALORIES 223; PROTEIN 6g; CARBOHYDRATES 33g; TOTAL FAT 8.5g; SATURATED FAT 0.7g; SODIUM 79mg; FIBER 6.9g; BETA-CAROTENE 10471ug; VITAMIN C 61mg; CALCIUM 130mg; IRON 2.7mg; FOLATE 92ug; MAGNESIUM 95mg; ZINC 1.2mg; SELENIUM 4.5ug

VEGETABLE TAGINE

Serves: 4

INGREDIENTS

1/2 cup water

1 large onion, chopped

2 carrots, chopped

1 red bell pepper, chopped

1 zucchini, small dice

1 clove garlic, minced

1/2 teaspoon cinnamon

1/2 teaspoon curry

1/2 teaspoon turmeric

1 1/2 cups diced tomatoes
or 1 (15 ounce) can no-salt-added or low sodium diced tomatoes

2 cups no-salt-added or low sodium vegetable stock

1/2 cup dried unsulfured apricots, soaked for 20 minutes
in 1/2 cup hot water

1/4 cup raisins

1 tablespoon lemon juice

1 1/2 cups cooked chickpeas
or 1 (15 ounce) can, no-salt-added or low sodium, drained

2 tablespoons fresh minced cilantro or parsley

DIRECTIONS

Heat water in saucepan over medium heat. Add onion, carrots and red pepper. Cover pan and cook for about 5 minutes. Add zucchini, garlic, cinnamon, turmeric, tomatoes, and vegetable stock and bring to a boil. Reduce heat to low and simmer for 25 minutes or until vegetables are tender. Drain apricots, reserving soaking liquid and chop. Add apricots, soaking liquid, raisins, lemon zest and chickpeas to vegetable mixture and cook 5 more minutes. Stir in cilantro or parsley and serve.

Note: Though the word tagine refers to the cone-shaped cooking vessel that the dish is traditionally made in, it has also come to refer to a Moroccan-style stew.

PER SERVING: CALORIES 242; PROTEIN 12g; CARBOHYDRATES 48g; TOTAL FAT 2.9g; SATURATED FAT 0.5g; SODIUM 77mg; FIBER 9.8g; BETA-CAROTENE 3816ug; VITAMIN C 63mg; CALCIUM 89mg; IRON 3.5mg; FOLATE 159ug; MAGNESIUM 67mg; ZINC 1.6mg; SELENIUM 3.1ug

NON-VEGAN DISHES

GARDEN EGGS AND TOFU WITH SALSA

Serves: 3

INGREDIENTS

- 1/2 medium onion, diced
- 1 medium zucchini, grated
- 1 carrot, grated
- 2 cups chopped Swiss chard or spinach
- 1/2 medium tomato, diced
- 2 cloves garlic, pressed
- 2 teaspoons herbes de Provence (dried French herbs)
- 1 cup firm tofu
- 1/8 teaspoon curry powder, or more to taste
- 3 large eggs, beaten
- 1/4 cup prepared low sodium salsa
- 1 ounce non-dairy mozzarella-type cheese substitute, grated
- 6 (100% whole grain) tortillas, if desired

DIRECTIONS

In a large sauté pan, heat 1/8 cup water and water sauté the onion, zucchini, carrot, and Swiss chard for about 2 minutes. Add the tomato, garlic, and herbs. Cook, stirring for about 2 minutes, until the vegetables begin to soften.

Squeeze water out of tofu and crumble.

Scatter the tofu over the vegetables and sprinkle with curry powder.

Mix with vegetables and cook over high heat until water is cooked away.

Reduce the heat to low and stir in the eggs, mixing well so the vegetables and tofu bind with the eggs. Continue stirring, until the eggs are cooked.

Top with salsa and grated cheese substitute. May be served on whole grain tortillas.

PER SERVING: CALORIES 261; PROTEIN 24g; CARBOHYDRATES 17g; TOTAL FAT 13.4g; SATURATED FAT 2.8g; CHOLESTEROL 211mg; SODIUM 291mg; FIBER 4.8g; BETA-CAROTENE 2776ug; VITAMIN C 26mg; CALCIUM 670mg; IRON 4.7mg; FOLATE 93ug; MAGNESIUM 120mg; ZINC 2.6mg; SELENIUM 33.2ug

MEDITERRANEAN FISH STEW

Serves: 4

INGREDIENTS

2 red bell peppers, sliced

2 medium onions, sliced

1 medium eggplant, cut into 1-inch pieces

2 medium zucchini, cut into 1-inch pieces

1 cup sliced mushrooms

6 medium tomatoes, chopped

2 cloves garlic, finely chopped

1 teaspoon Herbes de Provence

1/4 teaspoon black pepper

1/2 pound firm fish fillets, cut into 1-inch pieces
(such as halibut, bass, salmon)

2 tablespoons fresh chopped parsley

1 tablespoon fresh lemon juice

DIRECTIONS

Heat 1/8 cup water in a large pan. Add the bell peppers and onions and cook for 3 minutes, add the eggplant, zucchini and mushrooms and continue cooking for another 6-8 minutes or until tender, adding more water if necessary to keep from sticking.

Add the tomatoes, garlic, Herbes de Provence and black pepper and simmer on low heat for 4 minutes.

Add the fish to the stew and mix in gently. Cover and simmer on low heat for 8-10 minutes, stirring occasionally.

Before serving, stir in parsley and lemon juice.

PER SERVING: CALORIES 192; PROTEIN 23g; CARBOHYDRATES 29g; TOTAL FAT 2.5g; SATURATED FAT 0.4g; CHOLESTEROL 18.1mg; SODIUM 60mg; FIBER 10.7g; BETA-CAROTENE 2045ug; VITAMIN C 129mg; CALCIUM 102mg; IRON 3mg; FOLATE 139ug; MAGNESIUM 121mg; ZINC 1.5mg; SELENIUM 24.1ug

CREOLE CHICKEN AND SPINACH

Serves: 4

INGREDIENTS

8 ounces skinless, boneless organic chicken breasts, sliced thinly crosswise

1 cup chopped celery

1 1/2 cups chopped fresh tomatoes, or canned low sodium or no-salt-added diced tomatoes

10 ounces frozen spinach

1 large green pepper, chopped

1/2 cup chopped onion

4 cloves garlic, minced

1 cup low sodium chili sauce

1 tablespoon chopped fresh basil or 1 teaspoon dried

1 teaspoon chili powder or more to taste

1 tablespoon chopped fresh parsley or 1 teaspoon dried

1/4 teaspoon dried crushed red pepper

2 cups cooked brown rice and/or wild rice

DIRECTIONS

Cook chicken strips in a lightly oiled skillet, turning occasionally, for 3-5 minutes until no longer pink.

Add remaining ingredients except for rice, bring to a boil and reduce heat to medium. Simmer covered for 10 minutes or until vegetables are tender.

Serve over brown and or wild rice.

PER SERVING: CALORIES 293; PROTEIN 23g; CARBOHYDRATES 51g; TOTAL FAT 2.7g; SATURATED FAT 0.5g; CHOLESTEROL 34.2mg; SODIUM 140mg; FIBER 6.2g; BETA-CAROTENE 5565ug; VITAMIN C 62mg; CALCIUM 166mg; IRON 3.3mg; FOLATE 128ug; MAGNESIUM 133mg; ZINC 1.7mg; SELENIUM 25.8ug

SALMON AND VEGETABLES IN A PACKET

Serves: 4

INGREDIENTS

8 ounces salmon fillets or steaks divided into 4 pieces

freshly ground pepper

1 teaspoon freshly grated ginger root

juice of 1 lemon

3 ripe tomatoes, chopped

2 medium zucchini, chopped

2 cups sliced mushrooms

2 medium red onions, thinly sliced

2 cloves garlic, minced or pressed

4 cups coarsely chopped mustard greens or Swiss Chard

4 sheets aluminum foil, 12 X 24 inches

small amount of olive oil or olive oil cooking spray

DIRECTIONS

Preheat the oven to 450° F.

Place the salmon fillets in a glass baking dish and add pepper, grated ginger and lemon juice.

In a large bowl, mix tomatoes, zucchini, mushrooms, red onion and garlic.

Fold each piece of foil over to make a square of double thickness. Brush the center portion of each square with a small amount of olive oil.

On each square, place 1 cup chopped mustard greens, one salmon fillet and one quarter of the tomato/vegetable mixture.

Fold the foil into airtight packets. Bake for 20 minutes. Carefully avoiding the steam that will be released, open and packet and check that fish is cooked.

To serve, open the foil and transfer contents to a plate or bowl.

PER SERVING: CALORIES 226; PROTEIN 30g; CARBOHYDRATES 12g; TOTAL FAT 7.2g; SATURATED FAT 1.5g; CHOLESTEROL 51mg; SODIUM 78mg; FIBER 4.1g; BETA-CAROTENE 3864ug; VITAMIN C 65mg; CALCIUM 122mg; IRON 2.1mg; FOLATE 153ug; MAGNESIUM 76mg; ZINC 1.1mg; SELENIUM 46.7ug

SCRAMBLED VEGGIES AND EGGS

Serves: 2

INGREDIENTS

2 eggs

2 tablespoons unsweetened soy, hemp or almond milk

1/2 medium bell pepper, diced

2 green onions, chopped

1 cup diced fresh tomatoes

1 cup diced fresh mushrooms

1 tablespoon Dr. Fuhrman's VegiZest
or other no salt seasoning blend, adjusted to taste

1 teaspoon Spike or other no salt seasoning

4 ounces spinach, coarsely chopped

DIRECTIONS

Beat eggs with soy milk.

In 1/8 cup water, sauté the peppers, onions, tomatoes, mushrooms, VegiZest, and Spike until vegetables are tender. Add spinach to wilt.

Cook most water out of vegetables, then add eggs and scramble until cooked through.

PER SERVING: CALORIES 131; PROTEIN 13g; CARBOHYDRATES 11g; TOTAL FAT 5.8g; SATURATED FAT 1.7g; CHOLESTEROL 211mg; SODIUM 151mg; FIBER 3.3g; BETA-CAROTENE 4203ug; VITAMIN C 52mg; CALCIUM 108mg; IRON 3.7mg; FOLATE 163ug; MAGNESIUM 70mg; ZINC 1.3mg; SELENIUM 21.7ug

TURKEY SPINACH BURGERS

Serves: 5

INGREDIENTS

1 pound ground turkey breast

10 ounces frozen, chopped spinach, defrosted and drained

1/4 cup dried bread crumbs

1/4 cup chopped onion

2 tablespoons chopped fresh parsley

1 1/2 tablespoons vegan Worcestershire sauce

1 teaspoon hot sauce

DIRECTIONS

Combine the ground turkey, spinach, bread crumbs, onions, parsley, Worcestershire sauce, and hot sauce in a large bowl. Mix well.

Divide turkey mixture into 5 equal portions and form into patties.

Coat grill rack or broiler pan with cooking spray.

Grill or broil until nicely browned on both sides and cooked through, about 7 minutes per side.

PER SERVING: CALORIES 181; PROTEIN 19g; CARBOHYDRATES 8g; TOTAL FAT 8.2g; SATURATED FAT 2.2g; CHOLESTEROL 71.7mg; SODIUM 243mg; FIBER 2.2g; BETA-CAROTENE 4068ug; VITAMIN C 18mg; CALCIUM 119mg; IRON 2.9mg; FOLATE 90ug; MAGNESIUM 63mg; ZINC 2.1mg; SELENIUM 22.3ug

TURKEY-VEGETABLE MEATLOAF

Serves: 8

INGREDIENTS

2 pounds ground turkey

1 cup quick oats (not instant)

10 ounces frozen chopped spinach, thawed and drained

1 large carrot, grated

1 medium green bell pepper, chopped

1 medium onion, chopped

2 eggs

2 large cloves garlic, minced

6 tablespoons ketchup, low sodium

2 tablespoons vegan Worcestershire sauce

1 tablespoon chopped fresh basil

1 teaspoon Dijon mustard

1 teaspoon Italian herb seasoning

1/2 teaspoon marjoram

1/4 teaspoon black pepper

1 1/2 cups diced tomatoes
or 1 (15 ounce) can no-salt-added or low sodium diced tomatoes, drained

1 tablespoon low sodium ketchup

DIRECTIONS

Preheat oven to 350° F.

Mix ground turkey and oats together. Add remaining ingredients except for half of the tomatoes and ketchup. Mix well to combine.

Shape into loaf and place in a large loaf pan or spread in a tube pan.

Top with remaining tomatoes mixed with 1 tablespoon of ketchup.

Bake for 1 hour 15 minutes until meat is cooked through.

PER SERVING: CALORIES 320; PROTEIN 29g; CARBOHYDRATES 26g; TOTAL FAT 12.4g; SATURATED FAT 3.2g; CHOLESTEROL 142.5mg; SODIUM 230mg; FIBER 4.9g; BETA-CAROTENE 3539ug; VITAMIN C 24mg; CALCIUM 113mg; IRON 3.9mg; FOLATE 90ug; MAGNESIUM 102mg; ZINC 3.5mg; SELENIUM 32.7ug

VEGETABLE OMELET

Serves: 2

INGREDIENTS

1 medium onion, diced

1 medium green or red bell peppers, seeded and diced

1 1/2 cups chopped shiitake mushrooms,

1 cup diced fresh tomato

1/4 teaspoon dried basil

4 eggs, beaten

black pepper, to taste

DIRECTIONS

Lightly wipe a skillet with olive oil. Sauté the onion, bell pepper, mushrooms and tomato over medium heat for 10 minutes, or until tender. Add the basil and eggs and cook over medium-high heat until done, about 8 minutes, turning over with a spatula halfway through cooking. Sprinkle with black pepper, if desired.

PER SERVING: CALORIES 239; PROTEIN 19g; CARBOHYDRATES 22g; TOTAL FAT 10.6g; SATURATED FAT 3.2g; CHOLESTEROL 423mg; SODIUM 163mg; FIBER 4.4g; BETA-CAROTENE 1392ug; VITAMIN C 96mg; CALCIUM 105mg; IRON 3.1mg; FOLATE 134ug; MAGNESIUM 49mg; ZINC 1.9mg; SELENIUM 37.1ug

DESSERTS

APPLE SURPRISE

Serves: 6

INGREDIENTS

1 cup raisins

1/4 cup water

8 apples, peeled, cored and diced

1/2 cup chopped walnuts

4 tablespoons ground flax seeds

1 tablespoon cinnamon

DIRECTIONS

Place raisins in bottom of pot and cover with 1/4 cup water.

Place diced apples on top. Cover and steam over very low heat for 7 minutes.

Transfer apple/raisin mixture to a bowl and mix well with remaining ingredients.

Note: This recipe keeps well in the refrigerator for several days.

PER SERVING: CALORIES 260; PROTEIN 7g; CARBOHYDRATES 48g; TOTAL FAT 8.8g; SATURATED FAT 0.8g; SODIUM 7mg; FIBER 7.9g; BETA-CAROTENE 51ug; VITAMIN C 10mg; CALCIUM 59mg; IRON 1.7mg; FOLATE 21ug; MAGNESIUM 51mg; ZINC 0.7mg; SELENIUM 1.8ug

BANANA OAT BARS

Serves: 8

INGREDIENTS

2 cups quick-cooking rolled oats (not instant)

1/2 cup shredded unsweetened coconut

1/2 cup raisins or chopped dates

1/4 cup chopped walnuts

2 large ripe bananas, mashed

3/4 cup finely chopped apple

DIRECTIONS

Preheat oven to 350° F. Mix all the ingredients in a large bowl until well combined. Press into a 9-by-9-inch baking pan and bake for 30 minutes. Cool on a wire rack. When cool, cut into squares or bars.

PER SERVING: CALORIES 247; PROTEIN 8g; CARBOHYDRATES 41g; TOTAL FAT 6.9g; SATURATED FAT 2.2g; SODIUM 3mg; FIBER 5.9g; BETA-CAROTENE 8ug; VITAMIN C 3mg; CALCIUM 31mg; IRON 2.3mg; FOLATE 33ug; MAGNESIUM 87mg; ZINC 1.8mg; SELENIUM 11ug

BANANA WALNUT ICE CREAM

Serves: 2

INGREDIENTS

2 ripe bananas, frozen*

1/3 cup vanilla soy, hemp or almond milk

2 tablespoons chopped walnuts

DIRECTIONS

Blend all ingredients together in high powered blender until smooth and creamy.

* *Freeze ripe bananas at least 12 hours in advance. To freeze bananas, peel, cut in thirds and wrap tightly in plastic wrap.*

PER SERVING: CALORIES 174; PROTEIN 4g; CARBOHYDRATES 30g; TOTAL FAT 5.9g; SATURATED FAT 0.7g; SODIUM 23mg; FIBER 4.1g; BETA-CAROTENE 178ug; VITAMIN C 10mg; CALCIUM 28mg; IRON 1mg; FOLATE 37ug; MAGNESIUM 53mg; ZINC 0.6mg; SELENIUM 3.5ug

BLUEBERRY BANANA COBBLER

Serves: 2

INGREDIENTS

1 banana

1 cup frozen blueberries

1/4 cup old fashioned rolled oats

1 tablespoon dried currants

1/8 teaspoon vanilla

2 tablespoons chopped raw almonds

2 tablespoons unsweetened, shredded coconut

1/4 teaspoon cinnamon

DIRECTIONS

Combine banana, berries, oats, currents and vanilla in a microwave safe dish. Microwave for 2 minutes. Top with almonds, coconut and cinnamon and microwave for 1 minute. Serve warm.

PER SERVING: CALORIES 157; PROTEIN 2g; CARBOHYDRATES 28g; TOTAL FAT 5.3g; SATURATED FAT 1.8g; SODIUM 3mg; FIBER 5.2g; BETA-CAROTENE 39ug; VITAMIN C 8mg; CALCIUM 32mg; IRON 0.9mg; FOLATE 21ug; MAGNESIUM 39mg; ZINC 0.4mg; SELENIUM 1.4ug

BLUEVADO PIE

Serves: 8

INGREDIENTS

CRUST:

   10 date/coconut rolls (remove almonds)

   1 1/2 cups Familia, original Swiss baby muesli,
   no-added-sugar (found in supermarkets)

FILLING:

   10 ounces frozen blueberries

   10 dates, pitted and chopped

   4-5 bananas

   1 ripe avocado, peeled and pitted

   1 teaspoon unsweetened shredded coconut

DIRECTIONS

   For crust:

   In a bowl, thoroughly blend the date/coconut rolls and muesli. Transfer
   mixture to pie plate, pressing down to make pie crust.

   For filling:

   In a high powered blender, blend all filling ingredients, except for coconut,
   until smooth.

   Pour into the pie crust. Sprinkle with coconut.

   Cover and freeze for at least 3 hours before serving.

PER SERVING: CALORIES 264; PROTEIN 4g; CARBOHYDRATES 53g; TOTAL FAT 5.8g; SATURATED FAT 1.1g;
SODIUM 14mg; FIBER 8.2g; BETA-CAROTENE 47ug; VITAMIN C 13mg; CALCIUM 57mg; IRON 1.1mg;
FOLATE 35ug; MAGNESIUM 108mg; ZINC 0.8mg; SELENIUM 5.2ug

CHOCOLATE DIP

Serves: 8

INGREDIENTS

1 1/2 cups whole raw almonds or raw cashews

3/4 cup vanilla soy, hemp or almond milk

2 cups baby spinach

2 cups frozen strawberries or blueberries

2/3 cup dates, pitted

3 tablespoons natural, non-alkalized cocoa powder

2 tablespoons Goji berries, if desired

1 teaspoon vanilla extract

1/2 raw beet or 2 tablespoons beet powder, to adjust color

DIRECTIONS

Blend nuts and soy milk until smooth. Add remaining ingredients and blend again.

May be eaten as a pudding or used as a dip for fresh fruit and vegetables.

PER SERVING: CALORIES 193; PROTEIN 8g; CARBOHYDRATES 12g; TOTAL FAT 14.5g; SATURATED FAT 1.3g; SODIUM 31mg; FIBER 4.8g; BETA-CAROTENE 517ug; VITAMIN C 18mg; CALCIUM 84mg; IRON 2.1mg; FOLATE 39ug; MAGNESIUM 101mg; ZINC 1.2mg; SELENIUM 2.5ug

CHOCOLATE CHERRY SORBET

Serves: 2

INGREDIENTS

1/2 cup vanilla soy, hemp or almond milk

1 tablespoon natural, non-alkalized cocoa powder

4 dates, pitted

1 1/2 cups frozen dark sweet cherries

DIRECTIONS

Blend all ingredients together in a high powered blender or food processor until smooth and creamy. If using a regular blender, only add half the cherries, blend until smooth, then add remaining cherries and continue to blend.

Note: You can use berries or banana instead of cherries. Freeze ripe bananas at least 12 hours in advance. To freeze, peel into thirds, and wrap tightly in plastic wrap.

PER SERVING: CALORIES 109; PROTEIN 4g; CARBOHYDRATES 23g; TOTAL FAT 1.7g; SATURATED FAT 0.4g; SODIUM 34mg; FIBER 4.1g; BETA-CAROTENE 263ug; VITAMIN C 8mg; CALCIUM 41mg; IRON 1.4mg; FOLATE 15ug; MAGNESIUM 41mg; ZINC 0.5mg; SELENIUM 3.3ug

DR. FUHRMAN'S BANANA OAT COOKIES

Makes 14 cookies

INGREDIENTS

1/2 cup raisins or chopped dates

2 medium bananas, mashed

1 1/2 cups old fashioned oats

1/3 cup chopped walnuts or almonds

1/4 cup unsweetened, shredded coconut

1 teaspoon vanilla

1/8 teaspoon cinnamon

100% fruit spread, any flavor, if desired

DIRECTIONS

Add 2 tablespoons water to dates or raisins and soak for 30 minutes.

Preheat oven to 325° F.

Combine the mashed bananas and the oats. Add the nuts, coconut, vanilla, cinnamon, and the soaked dates or raisins. Mix well.

Drop by tablespoons onto a non-stick cookie sheet. If desired, flatten a little and make an indentation into the center of the cookie. Add the fruit spread.

Bake for 13 minutes or until golden brown.

PER SERVING: CALORIES 413; PROTEIN 12g; CARBOHYDRATES 72g; TOTAL FAT 10.6g; SATURATED FAT 1.4g; SODIUM 2mg; FIBER 10g; BETA-CAROTENE 38ug; VITAMIN C 5mg; CALCIUM 60mg; IRON 3.4mg; FOLATE 58ug; MAGNESIUM 148mg; ZINC 2.8mg; SELENIUM 16.1ug

FROZEN BANANA FLUFF

Serves: 2

INGREDIENTS

1/4 cup vanilla soy, hemp or almond milk

2 ripe bananas, frozen*

dash vanilla extract

2 tablespoons ground flax seeds

DIRECTIONS

Place the soy milk in the food processor, with the S blade in place.
Turn the machine on and drop in small slices of the frozen bananas, one by one. Add vanilla and combine until smooth and creamy.

Sprinkle ground flaxseeds on top, if desired.

* *Freeze ripe bananas at least 12 hours in advance. To freeze bananas, peel, cut in thirds, and wrap tightly in plastic wrap.*

PER SERVING: CALORIES 158; PROTEIN 4g; CARBOHYDRATES 30g; TOTAL FAT 3.9g; SATURATED FAT 0.5g; SODIUM 20mg; FIBER 5.4g; BETA-CAROTENE 141ug; VITAMIN C 10mg; CALCIUM 35mg; IRON 1mg; FOLATE 34ug; MAGNESIUM 67mg; ZINC 0.6mg; SELENIUM 4.4ug

HEALTHY CHOCOLATE CAKE

Serves: 12

INGREDIENTS

CAKE:

> 1 2/3 cups whole wheat flour
>
> 1 teaspoon baking powder
>
> 3 teaspoons baking soda
>
> 3 cups dates, pitted, divided
>
> 1 cup pineapple chunks in own juice, drained
>
> 1 banana
>
> 1 cup unsweetened applesauce
>
> 1 cup shredded beets
>
> 3/4 cup shredded carrots
>
> 1/2 cup shredded zucchini
>
> 4 tablespoons natural, non-alkalized cocoa powder
>
> 1/2 cup dried currants
>
> 1 cup chopped walnuts
>
> 1 1/2 cups water
>
> 2 teaspoons vanilla extract

CHOCOLATE NUT ICING:

> 1 cup raw macadamia nuts or raw cashews
>
> 1 cup vanilla soy, hemp or almond milk
>
> 2/3 cup dates, pitted
>
> 1/3 cup hazelnuts
>
> 2 tablespoons natural, non-alkalized cocoa powder
>
> 1 teaspoon vanilla extract

DIRECTIONS

Preheat oven to 350° F.

Mix flour, baking powder, and baking soda in a small bowl. Set aside.

In blender or food processor, puree 3 cups of the dates, pineapple, banana, and applesauce.

Slice remaining 1/2 cup dates into 1/2 inch thick pieces. In large bowl, mix sliced dates, beets, carrots, zucchini, cocoa powder, currants, walnuts, water, vanilla and flour mixture.

Add the blended mixture and mix well. Spread in a 9.5" X 13.5" nonstick baking pan.

Bake for 1 hour or until a toothpick inserted into the center comes out clean.

ICING:

Using a high powered blender*, combine all icing ingredients until smooth and creamy. Place a dollop over warm cake and serve. If desired, you may spread on cooled cake instead.

* A food processor may be used to combine icing ingredients but the icing will not be as smooth.

PER SERVING: CALORIES 454; PROTEIN 10g; CARBOHYDRATES 81g; TOTAL FAT 14.7g; SATURATED FAT 1.9g; SODIUM 347mg; FIBER 10.7g; BETA-CAROTENE 596ug; VITAMIN C 6mg; CALCIUM 86mg; IRON 3.4mg; FOLATE 60ug; MAGNESIUM 130mg; ZINC 2mg; SELENIUM 17ug

JENNA'S PEACH FREEZE

Serves: 2

INGREDIENTS

1 ripe banana, frozen*

3 peaches or nectarines, peeled and pitted

2 medjool dates, or 4 deglet noor dates, pitted

1/4 cup vanilla soy, hemp or almond milk

1 teaspoon vanilla extract

1/8 teaspoon cinnamon

DIRECTIONS

Blend all the ingredients in a high powered blender until smooth and creamy.

Freeze ripe bananas at least 24 hours in advance. To freeze, peel, cut into thirds, and wrap tightly in plastic wrap.

* Freeze ripe bananas at least 12 hours in advance. To freeze bananas, peel, cut in thirds, and wrap tightly in plastic wrap.

PER SERVING: CALORIES 179; PROTEIN 4g; CARBOHYDRATES 42g; TOTAL FAT 1.2g; SATURATED FAT 0.2g; SODIUM 18mg; FIBER 5.5g; BETA-CAROTENE 365ug; VITAMIN C 15mg; CALCIUM 32mg; IRON 1.1mg; FOLATE 26ug; MAGNESIUM 44mg; ZINC 0.5mg; SELENIUM 2.7ug

ORANGE GOJI BARS

Serves: 8

INGREDIENTS

1 cup old fashioned oats

1 cup chopped walnuts

1 cup dates, pitted

1/2 cup raisins

1 cup unsulphured dried apricots

1 cup Goji berries*

2 tablespoons unhulled sesame seeds

1 teaspoon dried organic orange zest

1 teaspoon water

DIRECTIONS

In a food processor, process oats until finely chopped, then add walnuts and process until chopped but not a powder. Remove to a mixing bowl.

Place dates, raisins, apricots, and Goji berries in food processor. Process until the mass forms one large ball.

Turn into mixing bowl and add sesame seeds, orange zest, and water along with the oat mixture and knead by hand until thoroughly combined.

Press into an 8 X 11 1/2-inch baking dish and cut into 12 bars.

---

* Goji berries are burnt-red in color and about the size of a raisin. They taste like a cross between a raisin, a cranberry, and a cherry. They are slightly sweet and tart. Dried blueberries or cherries may be substituted.

PER SERVING: CALORIES 353; PROTEIN 8g; CARBOHYDRATES 54g; TOTAL FAT 14.5g; SATURATED FAT 1.6g; SODIUM 6mg; FIBER 6.7g; BETA-CAROTENE 252ug; VITAMIN C 1mg; CALCIUM 123mg; IRON 3.3mg; FOLATE 37ug; MAGNESIUM 98mg; ZINC 1.9mg; SELENIUM 6.5ug

PEACH SORBET

Serves: 4

INGREDIENTS

1 pound frozen peaches

1/4 cup soy, hemp or almond milk

4 dates, pitted

DIRECTIONS

Blend ingredients until smooth in food processor or high powered blender.

PER SERVING: CALORIES 138; PROTEIN 2g; CARBOHYDRATES 34g; TOTAL FAT 0.5g; SATURATED FAT 0.1g; SODIUM 15mg; FIBER 2.9g; BETA-CAROTENE 215ug; VITAMIN C 107mg; CALCIUM 12mg; IRON 0.7mg; FOLATE 7ug; MAGNESIUM 13mg; ZINC 0.1mg; SELENIUM 1.4ug

POACHED PEARS WITH RASPBERRY SAUCE

Serves: 2

INGREDIENTS

2 pears

1 teaspoon lemon juice

2/3 cup frozen red raspberries, thawed

1 medjool date, pitted

DIRECTIONS

Peel the pears and leave the stems attached. Drizzle with lemon juice.

Microwave for 4 minutes. Do not drain.

Blend raspberries and the date in a high powered blender until smooth. Mix with cooking liquid.

Top pears with raspberry sauce.

PER SERVING: CALORIES 151; PROTEIN 1g; CARBOHYDRATES 40g; TOTAL FAT 0.5g; SODIUM 2mg; FIBER 8.6g; BETA-CAROTENE 37ug; VITAMIN C 19mg; CALCIUM 33mg; IRON 0.7mg; FOLATE 22ug; MAGNESIUM 27mg; ZINC 0.4mg; SELENIUM 0.3ug

RED VELVET SORBET

Serves: 4

INGREDIENTS

4 large ripe bananas, frozen*

10 ounces frozen raspberries

2 tablespoons natural, non-alkalized cocoa powder

4-5 dates, pitted, chopped

DIRECTIONS

Blend all ingredients in a high powered blender until creamy. Refreeze briefly (3-5 minutes).

* *Freeze ripe bananas at least 24 hours in advance. To freeze bananas, peel, cut in thirds, and wrap tightly in plastic wrap.*

PER SERVING: CALORIES 171; PROTEIN 3g; CARBOHYDRATES 43g; TOTAL FAT 1.2g; SATURATED FAT 0.4g; SODIUM 3mg; FIBER 9.2g; BETA-CAROTENE 40ug; VITAMIN C 29mg; CALCIUM 30mg; IRON 1.2mg; FOLATE 41ug; MAGNESIUM 63mg; ZINC 0.7mg; SELENIUM 1.9ug

STRAWBERRY PINEAPPLE SORBET

Serves: 2

INGREDIENTS

1 (10-ounce) bag frozen strawberries

1/2 cup orange juice or soy, hemp or almond milk

4 slices dried unsweetened, unsulphured pineapple

1 cup fresh organic strawberries, sliced

DIRECTIONS

Blend all ingredients except fresh strawberries in a high-powered blender.

Pour into sorbet glasses and top with sliced fresh strawberries.

PER SERVING: CALORIES 150; PROTEIN 2g; CARBOHYDRATES 38g; TOTAL FAT 0.5g; SODIUM 12mg; FIBER 4.9g; BETA-CAROTENE 64ug; VITAMIN C 132mg; CALCIUM 49mg; IRON 1.5mg; FOLATE 60ug; MAGNESIUM 32mg; ZINC 0.3mg; SELENIUM 1.3ug

SUMMER FRUIT PIE

Serves: 8

INGREDIENTS

PIE SHELL:

> 1 cup almonds
>
> 1 cup dates, pitted
>
> 2 tablespoons unsweetened, shredded coconut

PIE FILLING:

> 3 bananas, sliced
>
> 1 teaspoon lemon juice
>
> 2 kiwis, sliced
>
> 1 quart organic strawberries, sliced,
>
> 1 pint blueberries,
>
> 1/2 cup vanilla soy, hemp or almond milk
>
> 1/2 bag frozen strawberries or 1 pint fresh organic strawberries
>
> 2 dates, pitted

DIRECTIONS

Make pie shell by placing almonds in a food processor or high powered blender and processing until very fine. Add dates and process until chopped and mixed well. Remove from food processor and hand knead with shredded coconut. Press mixture in a 9 inch pie plate to form shell.

To make the filling, spread bananas on the crust, pressing down slightly. Sprinkle lemon juice over the bananas. Place kiwis, strawberries and blueberries over the bananas. If desired, reserve some fruit to decorate top of pie.

Add the soy milk, frozen strawberries and dates in a blender and blend until smooth. Pour blended mixture over the fruit. Decorate with additional fruit as desired. Cover and freeze for at least two hours before serving.

PER SERVING: CALORIES 245; PROTEIN 9g; CARBOHYDRATES 47g; TOTAL FAT 6.8g; SATURATED FAT 0.6g; SODIUM 11mg; FIBER 8g; BETA-CAROTENE 101ug; VITAMIN C 76mg; CALCIUM 70mg; IRON 1.6mg; FOLATE 47ug; MAGNESIUM 75mg; ZINC 0.8mg; SELENIUM 2.7ug

VERY BERRY SORBET

Serves: 3

INGREDIENTS

1/2 package frozen peaches

1/2 package frozen mixed berries

1 cup soy, hemp or almond milk

1 banana

DIRECTIONS

Blend all ingredients in in a high powered blender until smooth and creamy.

PER SERVING: CALORIES 130; PROTEIN 2g; CARBOHYDRATES 33g; TOTAL FAT 0.5g; SATURATED FAT 0.1g; SODIUM 4mg; FIBER 3.8g; BETA-CAROTENE 153ug; VITAMIN C 40mg; CALCIUM 24mg; IRON 1.2mg; FOLATE 24ug; MAGNESIUM 28mg; ZINC 0.3mg; SELENIUM 1.1ug

WILD APPLE CRUNCH

Serves: 8

INGREDIENTS

6 apples, peeled and sliced

3/4 cup chopped walnuts

8 dates, pitted, chopped

1 cup dried currants or raisins

3/4 cup water

1/2 teaspoon cinnamon

1/4 teaspoon nutmeg

juice of 1 orange

DIRECTIONS

Preheat oven to 375° F.

Combine all ingredients except the orange juice. Place in an 8 X 8 inch baking pan and drizzle the orange juice on top.

Cover and bake for about one hour until all ingredients are soft, stirring occasionally.

Note: You can also simmer this in a covered pot for 30 minutes on top of the stove, stirring occasionally.

PER SERVING: CALORIES 207; PROTEIN 5g; CARBOHYDRATES 37g; TOTAL FAT 7.5g; SATURATED FAT 0.7g; SODIUM 4mg; FIBER 4.7g; BETA-CAROTENE 32ug; VITAMIN C 9mg; CALCIUM 33mg; IRON 0.9mg; FOLATE 19ug; MAGNESIUM 33mg; ZINC 0.5mg; SELENIUM 0.9ug

GLOSSARY

Acrylamides: Cancer-causing agents formed during high temperature cooking such as frying, baking, roasting, and grilling.

Advanced Glycation End Products (AGEs): The end products of a chain of chemical reactions in which a sugar molecule bonds to either a protein or lipid molecule. AGEs may be formed inside the body through cellular metabolism or externally by overcooking foods. AGE's increase when starchy foods are cooked at high temperatures in the absence of water. They have been implicated in the progression of Alzheimer's disease, cardiovascular disease, stroke, diabetes and other age related diseases.

ANDI (Aggregate Nutrient Density Index): Index developed by Joel Fuhrman, M.D. that assigns a score to a variety of foods based on how many nutrients they deliver to your body for each calorie consumed.

Angina: Chest pain due to a lack of blood and oxygen supply to the heart, generally due to coronary artery disease.

Angioplasty: A technique of mechanically widening a blood vessel that is narrowed or obstructed, typically as a result of atherosclerosis. The blood vessel is expanded by means of a balloon catheter which is inserted and then inflated to a fixed size.

Angiogenesis: The new growth of blood vessels from preexisting blood vessels. This is a normal process in growth and development, as well as in wound healing; however, it is also a fundamental step in the transition of tumors from a harmless state to a malignant (cancerous) state.

Antioxidant: A substance that protects cells against the effects of damaging free radicals by neutralizing or stabilizing them. Antioxidants are found in fruits, vegetables, nuts, seeds and grains.

Aromatase Inhibitor: A substance or drug that inhibits or slows the production or effects of the hormone estrogen. These drugs are often used in the treatment of estrogen-related cancers, such as breast or ovarian cancer. Natural foods such as mushrooms also act as aromatase inhibitors.

Arthritis: Acute or chronic inflammation of a joint, often accompanied by pain and structural changes and having diverse causes, as infection or injury.

Atherosclerosis: A condition in which fatty material collects along the walls of arteries, forming a thick and hardened plaque. This plaque reduces blood flow to the heart and may result in chest pain and cause heart attack or stroke.

Autoimmune Disease: A disease resulting from a disordered immune reaction in which antibodies are produced against one's own tissue. Examples include rheumatoid arthritis, lupus, multiple sclerosis, Crohn's disease, ulcerative colitis and psoriasis.

Blood Sugar: The quantity or percentage of glucose in the blood, normally tightly regulated by the human body. Blood sugar levels outside the normal range may be an indicator of a medical condition such as diabetes.

Cardiomyopathy: A disease that abnormally enlarges the heart muscle, leading to decreased function.

Coronary Heart Disease: Atherosclerotic disease of the coronary arteries that supply blood to fuel the heart's function.

Crohn's Disease: A form of inflammatory bowel disease and autoimmune disorder characterized by ongoing (chronic) inflammation of the gastrointestinal tract and causing abdominal pain and diarrhea, which can lead to narrowing of the bowel and even malnutrition.

Detoxification: The body's efforts to reduce its toxic load by changing irritants to a less harmful form or one that can be more readily eliminated, or the body's efforts to force the expulsion of such substances through channels of elimination, such as mucus, urine, or skin.

Dementia: Severe impairment or loss of intellectual capacity and personality integration, due to the loss of or damage to neurons in the brain.

DHA (docosahexaenoic acid): An omega-3 fatty acid important for normal brain function and the development of the nervous system. The body can manufacture DHA from alpha-linolenic acid, found in seeds and greens, or get it directly from certain fish, from an algae-derived supplement, or from a fish oil supplement.

Dyspepsia: Indigestion or impaired digestion; upset stomach.

EPA (eicosapentaenoic acid): An omega-3 fatty acid that has the ability to reduce inflammation, inhibit cancer development, and protect blood vessels. EPA can be obtained from fish, fish oils, or derived from specially grown algae or yeast.

Fibromyalgia: A syndrome characterized by fatigue and chronic pain in the muscles and in tissues surrounding the joints.

Flavonoid: A polyphenolic compound that is ubiquitous in nature. Over 4,000 flavonoids have been identified in colorful fruits and vegetables and are known to have antiviral, anti-allergic, anti-inflammatory, antitumor, and antioxidant activities.

Flexitarian: A person who eats mostly a vegetarian, plant-based diet but will occasionally eat animal products such as meat, poultry, or fish.

Free Radical: An atom or molecule with an odd number of electrons. The resulting "unpaired" electrons make the free radical reactive and unstable. Once formed, free radicals start a chain reaction that can damage important cellular components, such as DNA. Free radical damage can result in a variety of diseases and even cancers.

Gastric Bypass: A type of bariatric (weight loss) surgery that makes the stomach smaller and allows food to bypass part of the small intestine. Gastric bypass limits the amount of food that can be ingested and absorbed. It is conducted on obese patients who have been unable to lose weight through diet and exercise.

Glycemic Index: A measure of the effects of carbohydrates in food on blood sugar levels. It estimates how much each gram of available carbohydrate in a food raises a person's blood glucose level, relative to the consumption of glucose. Glucose has a glycemic index of 100, by definition and other foods have a lower value.

HDL Cholesterol: The cholesterol in high-density lipoproteins; the 'good' cholesterol; a high level in the blood is thought to lower the risk of coronary artery disease.

Hydrogenated Oil: An oil that has been chemically changed from a room-temperature liquid state into a solid. Hydrogenated oils contain trans fats.

Hypercholesterolemic: The presence of an excessive amount of cholesterol in the blood.

Hypertension: A term used to describe high blood pressure, the measurement of the force against the walls of your arteries as your heart pumps blood through your body.

Hypoglycemia: An abnormally low level of glucose in the blood. A common problem among diabetics from the over-use of medications when trying to control blood sugar levels.

Insulin-like Growth Factor 1 (IGF-1): A key contributor to brain development, muscle and bone growth and maintenance, body composition and sexual maturation. While crucial for growth and development, high levels of IGF-1 are strongly linked to cancer development and all-cause and cardiovascular mortality. High consumption of animal protein raises IGF-1 levels.

LDL Cholesterol: The cholesterol in low-density lipoproteins; the 'bad' cholesterol; a high level in the blood is thought to be related to various pathogenic conditions by accelerating atherosclerosis.

Lipids: A group of water-insoluble fatty substances that serve biological functions in the body: an expression to represent the group of lipoproteins affecting heart disease risk, such as cholesterol, triglycerides, and their component subtypes.

Lupus: An autoimmune disease that results in a variety of symptoms. Discoid lupus is limited to the skin and is characterized by a rash that appears on the face, neck and scalp and does not affect internal organs. Systemic lupus erythematosus (SLE) is more severe and can result in symptoms such as inflammation, swelling and damage to joints, kidneys, blood, the heart and lungs.

Macronutrients: The four major substances needed in relatively larger amounts by the body which include the fats, carbohydrates, and protein, which supply calories (energy) and are necessary for growth and normal function as well as water.

Micronutrients: Essential dietary elements required in small quantities for various bodily needs, but not a source of calories. Micronutrients include minerals, vitamins, and phytochemicals.

Nutritarian: A person who has a preference for an eating style high in micronutrients. The word was coined by Dr. Fuhrman.

Omega-3 Fatty Acid: A class of fatty acid that includes ALA (alpha-linolenic acid) from vegetables, seeds, and nuts, but also includes the longer-chain omega-3s, EPA and DHA, which are commonly found in fish oil (but which the body can manufacture from ALA). Omega-3 fatty acids confer a number health benefits and are necessary for optimal functioning of the immune system, brain, and cardiovascular system.

Osteoarthritis: A common joint disorder in which joints of the body are stiff or painful and difficult to move.

Osteoporosis: A common bone disease in which bones become thinner and less dense over time.

Peripheral Vascular Disease (PVP): A disease or disorder of the circulatory system outside of the brain or heart. PVP can result from atherosclerosis and causes acute or chronic ischemia or lack of blood supply. Also called arteriosclerosis or hardening of the arteries (outside of the coronary arteries).

Peristalsis: A series of organized muscle contractions that occur throughout the digestive tract that are part of the process that moves food through the digestive system.

Phytochemicals: Numerous newly discovered micronutrients present in plant foods with substantial ability to maximize the body's defenses against developing disease, including protection from toxins and carcinogens.

Pulmonary Embolism: A blockage of the main artery of the lung or one of its branches, usually by detached fragments of a clot from a leg or pelvic vein.

Retinopathy: Damage to the blood vessels of the retina of the eye that can eventually lead to blindness. Commonly seen as a complication of diabetes.

Sarcoidosis: An autoimmune disease characterized by the development and growth of tiny clumps of inflammatory cells in different areas of the body, most commonly the lungs, lymph nodes, eyes and skin.

Saturated Fat: A fat, most often of animal origin, having chains of fatty acids which are saturated (contain the maximum number hydrogen atoms). An excess of these fats in the diet tends to raise cholesterol levels in the bloodstream. Saturated fats are typically solid at room temperature.

Standard American Diet (SAD): A dietary habit chosen by many people in developed countries, especially America. It is characterized by high intakes of animal products, sweets, cooking oils, high-fat foods and processed foods. SAD is associated with heart disease and cancers.

N-Nitroso Compounds: Carcinogens synthesized during food processing. Found in high concentrations in cured meats, bacon, smoked fish and luncheon meats.

Trans Fats: Man-made or processed fats, made by a process called hydrogenation which produces a fat that is solid at room temperature and less likely to spoil. Raises LDL cholesterol more than any other type of fat.

Triglyceride: A substance formed in the body from fat in the diet. Triglycerides are the main fatty materials in the blood. Together with protein, they make up high and low-density lipoproteins (HDLs and LDLs). Excess increases risk of heart disease.

Ulcerative Colitis: An inflammatory bowel disease and autoimmune disorder that causes swelling, ulcerations and loss of function of the large intestine. Symptoms include abdominal pain, diarrhea and rectal bleeding.

Venous Thrombosis: A blood clot (thrombus) that forms within a vein. Deep venous thromboses form mainly in the large veins in the lower leg and thigh and can block blood flow. If the clot breaks off and moves through the bloodstream, it can get stuck in the brain, lungs, heart or other area, leading to severe damage.

REFERENCES

1. Fuhrman J, Sarter B, et al. Changing perceptions of hunger on a high nutrient density diet. Nutrition Journal 2010;9:51.

2. Svendsen M, Blomhoff R,Holme I, Tonstad S. The effect of an increased intake of vegetables and fruit on weight loss, blood pressure and antioxidant defense in subjects with sleep related breathing disorders. Euro J Cl in Nutr. 2007;61:1301–1311. Ello-Martin JA, Roe LS, Ledikwe JH, et al. Dietary energy density in the treatment of obesity: a year-long trial comparing 2 weight-loss diets. Am J Clin Nutr. 2007; 85(6):1465-1477. Howard BV, Manson JE, Stefanick ML, et al. Low-fat dietary pattern and weight change over 7 years: the Women's Health Initiative Dietary Modification Trial. JAMA. 2006; 295(1):39-49.

3. Bunyard LB, Dennis KE, Nicklas BJ. Dietary intake and changes in lipoprotein lipids in obese, postmenopausal women placed on an American Heart Association Step 1 diet. J Am Diet Assoc 2002 Jan;102(1):52-57.

4. Sharman MJ, Kraemer WJ, Love DM, et al. A ketogenic diet favorably affects serum biomarkers for cardiovascular disease in normal-weight men. J Nutr 2002 Jul;132(7):1879-1885.

5. Barnard ND, Scialli AR, Bertron P, et al. Effectiveness of a low-fat vegetarian diet in altering serum lipids in healthy premenopausal women. Am J Cardiol 2000 Apr 15;85(8):969-972.

6. Bemelmans WJ, Broer J, de Vries JH, et al. Impact of Mediterranean diet education versus posted leaflet on dietary habits and serum cholesterol in a high risk population for cardiovascular disease. Public Health Nutr. 2000 Sep;3(3):273-283.

7. Frolkis JP, Pearce GL, Nambi V, et al. Statins do not meet expectations for lowering low-density lipoprotein cholesterol levels when used in clinical practice. Am J Med 2002 Dec 1;113(8):625-629.

8. Jenkins DJ, Kendall CW, Popovich DG, et al. Effect of a very-high-fiber vegetable, fruit and nut diet on serum lipids and colonic function. Metabolism 2001 Apr;50(4):494-503.

9. Ward S, Lloyd JM, Pandor A, et al. A systematic review and economic evaluation of statins for the prevention of coronary events. Health Technol Assess. 2007;11(14):1-178.

10. Gardner CD, Coulston A, Chatterjee L, et al. The effect of a plant-based diet on plasma lipids in hypercholesterolemic adults: a randomized trial. Ann Intern Med. 2005;135(3):556-561.

11. Tucker KL, Hallfrisch J, Qiao N, et al. The combination of high fruit and vegetable and low saturated fat intakes is more protective against mortality in aging men than is either alone: the Baltimore Longitudinal Study of Aging. J Nutr. 2005;135(3):556-561.

12. Hu FB. Plant-based foods and prevention of cardiovascular disease: an overview. Am J Clin Nutr. 2003;78(3 Suppl):544S-551S.

13. Ornish D, Scherwitz L, Billings J, et al. Intensive Lifestyle Changes for Reversal of Coronary Heart Disease. JAMA. 1998; 280(23): 2001-2007.

14. Schauer PR, Burguera B, Ikramuddin S, et al. Effect of laparoscopic Roux-en Y gastric bypass on type 2 diabetes mellitus. Ann Surg. 2003;238(4):467- 484; discussion 84-85.

15. Harder H, Dinesen B, Astrup A. The effect of a rapid weight loss on lipid profile and glycemic control in obese type 2 diabetic patients. Int J Obes Relat Metab Disord. 2004;28(1):180-182.

16. Barnard ND, Cohen J, Jenkins DJ, et al. A low-fat vegan diet improves glycemic control and cardiovascular risk factors in a randomized clinical trial in individuals with type 2 diabetes. Diabetes Care. 2006;29(8):1777-1783. Ford ES, Mokdad AH. Fruit and vegetable consumption and diabetes mellitus incidence among U.S. adults. Prev Med 2001;32(1):33-39. Ford ES, Mokdad AH. Fruit and vegetable consumption and diabetes mellitus incidence among U.S. adults. Prev Med 2001;32(1):33-39. Montonen J, Knekt P, Harkanen T, et al. Dietary patterns and the incidence of Type 2 Diabetes. Am J Epidem 2004;161(3):219-227.

17. Fuhrman J, Sarter B, Calabro DJ. Brief case reports of medically supervised, water-only fasting associated with remission of autoimmune disease. Altern-Ther-Health-Med. 2002 Jul-Aug; 8(4):110-112.

18. NenonenM, Törrönen R, Häkkinen AS, et al. Antioxidants in vegan diet and rheumatic disorders. Toxicology. 2000;155(1-3):45-53. Müller H, de Toledo FW, Resch KL, et al. Fasting followed by vegetarian diet in patients with rheumatoid arthritis: a systematic review. Scand J Rheumatol. 2001;30(1):1- 10. McDougall J, Bruce B, Spiller G, et al. Effects of a very low-fat, vegan diet in subjects with rheumatoid arthritis. J Altern Complement Med. 2002;8(1):71-75. Darlington LG, Ramsey NW, Mansfield JR. Placebocontrolled, blind study of dietary manipulation therapy in rheumatoid arthritis. Lancet 1986;1(8475):236-238.

19. Liu RH. Potential synergy of phytochemicals in cancer prevention: mechanism of action. J Nutr. 2004;134(12 Suppl):3479S-3485S. Weiss JF, Landauer MR. Protection against ionizing radiation by antioxidant nutrients and phytochemicals. Toxicology 2003;189(1-2):1-20. Carratù B, Sanzini E. Biologically-active phytochemicals in vegetable food. Ann Ist Super Sanita. 2005; 41(1):7-16.

20. Hu FB. Plant-based foods and prevention of cardiovascular disease: an overview. Am J Clin Nutr. 2003 Sep;78(3 Suppl):544S-551S. Campbell TC, Parpia B, Chen J. Diet, lifestyle, and the etiology of coronary artery disease: the Cornell China study. Am J Cardiol 1998 Nov 26;82(10B):18T-21T. Fujimoto N, Matsubayashi K, Miyahara T, et al. The risk factors for ischemic heart disease in Tibetan highlanders. Jpn Heart J. 1989 Jan;30(1):27-34. Tatsukawa M, Sawayama Y, Maeda N, et al. Carotid atherosclerosis and cardiovascular risk factors: a comparison of residents of a rural area of Okinawa with residents of a typical suburban area of Fukuoka, Japan. Atherosclerosis 2004;172(2):337-343.

21. Hu FB, Willett WC. Optimal diets for prevention of coronary heart disease. JAMA 2002 Nov 27;288(20):2569-2578. Esselstyn CB. Resolving the Coronary Artery Disease Epidemic Through Plant-Based Nutrition. 2001 Autumn;4(4):171-177.

22. Gardner CD, Coulston A, Chatterjee L, et al. The effect of a plant-based diet on plasma lipids in hypercholesterolemic adults: a randomized trial. Ann Intern Med. 2005;142(9):725-733. Tucker KL, Hallfrisch J, Qiao N, et al. The combination of high fruit and vegetable and low saturated fat intakes is more protective against mortality in aging men than is either alone: the Baltimore Longitudinal Study of Aging. J Nutr. 2005;135(3):556-561.

23. Vasan RS, Beiser A, Seshadri S, et al. Residual lifetime risk for developing hypertension in middle-aged women and men: The Framingham Heart Study. JAMA 2002;287(8):1003-1010.

24. Black HR. The burden of cardiovascular disease: following the link from hypertension to myocardial infarction and heart failure. Am J Hypertens. 2003;16(9 Pt 2):4S-6S.

25. Freis ED. Salt, volume and the prevention of hypertension. Circulation 1976;54:589.

26. Ziegler RG, Hoover RN, Pike MC, et al. Migration Patterns and Breast Cancer Risk in Asian-American Women. J. Natl. Cancer Inst.1993;85:1819-1827.

27. Giles LC. Effect of social networks on 10 year survival in very old Australians: the Australian longitudinal study of aging. Journal of Epidemiology and Community Health July 2005;59(7):574-579.

28. Lea EJ, Crawford D, Worsley A. Consumers' readiness to eat a plant-based diet. European Journal of Clinical Nutrition 2006;60:342–351.

29. Mattson MP, Wan R. Beneficial effects of intermittent fasting and caloric restriction on the cardiovascular and cerebrovascular systems. J Nutr Biochem. 2005;16(3):129-137.

30. Bouchard C. The causes of obesity: advances in molecular biology but stagnation on the genetic front. Diabetologia 1996;39(12):1532-1533.

31. Weinsier RL, Krumdieck CL. Dairy foods and bone health: examination of the evidence. Am J Clin Nutr 2000;72:681–689.

32. Sellmeyer DE, Stone KL, Sebastian A, Cummings AR. A high ratio of dietary animal to vegetable protein increases the rate of bone loss and the risk of fracture in postmenopausal women, Am J Clin Nutr 2001; 73:118-22.

33. Sinnett PF, Whyte HM. Epidemiological studies in total highland population, Tukisenta, New Guinea. Cardiovascular disease and relevant clinical, electrocardiography, radiological and biochemical findings. J Chron Diseases 1973;26:265. Campbell TC, Parpia B, Chen J. Diet, lifestyle and the etiology of coronary artery disease: The Cornell China Study. Am J Card 1998;82(10B):18T-21T. Miller K. Lipid values in Kalahari Bushman. Arch Intern Med 1968;121:414. Breslow JL. Cardiovascular disease myths and facts. Cleve Clin J Med. 1998;65(6):286-287.

34. Commenges D, Scotet V, Renaud S, et al. Intake of flavonoids and risk of dementia. Eur J Epidemiol. 2000;16(4):357-363. Otsuka M, Yamaguchi K, Ueki A. Similarities and differences between Alzheimer's disease and vascular dementia from the viewpoint of nutrition. Ann NY Acad Sci. 2002;977:155-161. Nash DT, Fillit H. Cardiovascular disease risk factors and cognitive impairment. Am J Cardiol. 2006;97(8):1262-1265.

35. Golay A, Guy-Grand B. Are diets fattening? Ann Endocrinol 2002;63(6):2.

36. Maguire EA, Spiers HJ, Good CD, et al. Navigation expertise and the human hippocampus: a structural brain imaging analysis. Hippocampus. 2003;13(2):250-259.

37. He FJ, MacGregor GA. Blood pressure is the most important cause of death and disability in the world. European Heart Journal Supplements 2007;9:B23-B28.

38. Seals DR, Tanaka H, Clevenger CM, et al Blood pressure reductions with exercise and sodium restriction in postmenopausal women with elevated systolic pressure: role of arterial stiffness. J Am Coll Cardiol, 2001; 38:506-513

39. Cook NR, Cutler JA, Obarzanek E, et al. Long term effects of dietary sodium reduction on cardiovascular disease outcomes: observational follow-up of the trials of hypertension prevention (TOHP). BMJ 2007; 334(7599):885.

40. Tuomilehto J, Jousilahti P, Rastenyte D, et al. Urinary sodium excretion and cardiovascular mortality in Finland: a prospective study. Lancet 2001;357:848-851.

41. Tirschwell DL, Smith NL, Heckbert SR, et al. Association of cholesterol with stroke risk varies in stroke subtypes and patient subgroups. Neurology 2004;63(10):1868-1875.

42. Roberts JC, Moses C, Wilkins RH. Autopsy Studies in Atherosclerosis. I. Distribution and Severity of Atherosclerosis in Patients Dying without Morphologic Evidence of Atherosclerotic Catastrophe. Circulation 1959;20:511. Berenson GS, et al. Bogalusa Heart Study: A long-term community study of a rural biracial (black/white) population. Am J Med Sci 2001;322(5):267-274.

43. Huxley R, Lewington S, Clarke R. Cholesterol, coronary heart disease and stroke: a review of published evidence from observational studies and randomized controlled trials. Semin Vasc Med. 2002;2(3):315-323.

44. Hu FB, Manson JE, Willett WC. Types of dietary fat and risk of coronary heart disease: a critical review. J Am Coll Nutr. 2001;20(1):5-19.

45. Duwe AK, Fitch M, Ostwald R, et al. Depressed Natural Killer and Lecithin-Induced Cell-Mediated Cytotoxicity in Cholesterol-Fed Guinea Pigs. J Nat Cancer Inst 1984;72(2):333-338.

46. Composition of Foods - Raw-Processed-Prepared, Agriculture Handbook 8. Series and Supplements. United States Department of Agriculture, Human Nutrition Information Service, Minnesota Nutrition Data System (NDS) software, developed by the Nutrition Coordinating Center, University of Minnesota, Minneapolis, MN. Food Database version 5A, Nutrient Database version 20, USDA Nutrient Database for Standard Reference. Release 14 at www.nal.usda.gov.fnic

47. Okuyama H, Kobayashi T, Watanabe S. Dietary fatty acids—the N-6/N-3 balance and chronic elderly diseases. Excess linoleic acid and relative N-3 deficiency syndrome seen in Japan. Prog Lipid Res. 1996 Dec;35(4):409-457.

48. Itabe H. Oxidized Phospholipids as a New Landmark in Atherosclerosis. Prog Lipid Research 1998;37(2/3):181-207.

49. Tucker KL, Hallfrisch J, Qiao N, et al. The combination of high fruit and vegetable and low saturated fat intakes is more protective against mortality in aging men than is either alone: the Baltimore Longitudinal Study of Aging. J Nutr. 2005;135(3):556-561.

50. Fontana L, Wess EP, Villareal DT, et al. "Long-term effects of calorie or protein restriction on serum IGF-1 and IGFBP-3 concentration in humans." Aging Cell 2008;7(5)681-687. Fontana L. "The scientific basis of caloric restriction leading to longer life." Curr Opin Gastroenterol 2009;25(2):144-50.

51. Larsson SC, Rafter J, Holmberg L, et al. Red meat consumption and risk of cancers of the proximal colon, distal colon and rectum: the Swedish Mammography Cohort. Int J Cancer 2005; 113(5):829-834. Larsson SC, Håkanson N, Permert J, Wolk A. Meat, fish, poultry and egg consumption in relation to risk of pancreatic cancer: a prospective study. Int J Cancer 2006; 118(11):2866-2870.

52. Chao A, Thun JT, Connell CJ, et al. Meat Consumption and Risk of Colorectal Cancer JAMA 2005;293:172-182.

53. Sesink AL, Termont DS, Kleibeuker JH, Van derMcer R. Red meat and colon cancer: dietary haem-induced colonic cytotoxicity and epithelial hyperprolif-cration are inhibited by calcium. Carcinogenesis 2001;22(10):1653-1659. Hughes R, Cross AJ, Pollock JR, Bingham S. Dose-dependent effect of dietary meat on endogenous colonic N-nitrosation. Carcinogenesis 2001; 22(1):199-202.

54. Hightower JM, Moore D. Mercury levels in high-end consumers of fish. Environmental Health Perspectives 2003;111(4):604-608. Mahaffey KR, Clickner RP, Bodurow CC. Blood organic mercury and dietary mercury intake: National Health and Nutrition Examination Survey, 1999 and 2000. Env Health Persp 2004;112(5):562-570.

55. Hightower JM, Moore D. "Mercury levels in high-end consumers of fish." Env Health Persp 2003;111(4):604-608. Mahaffey KR, Clickner RP, Bodurow CC. "Blood organic mercury and dietary mercury intake: National Health and Nutrition Examination Survey, 1999 and 2000." Env Health Persp 2004;112(5):562-570.

56. Ma RW, Chapman K. "A systematic review of the effect of diet in prostate cancer and prevention and treatment." J hum Nutr Diet 2009 Jun;22(3):187-99;quiz 200-2. Epub 2009 April.

57. Cohen JM, Stampfer MJ, Giovannucci E, et al. "Plasma Insulin like growth factor-1and prostate caner risk: a prospective study." Science 1998(279):563-565.

58. Johnson K. "Dairy products linked to ovarian cancer risk." Family Practice News 2000 Jun 15:8.

59. Melita A, Jain AC, Mehta MC, Billie M. Caffeine and cardiac arrhythmias, An experimental study in dogs with review of literature. Acta Cardiol 1997;52(3):273-283. Nurminen MI, Niittymen L, Retterstol I, et al. Coffee, caffeine, and blood pressure: a critical review. Eur J Clin Nutr 1999;53(11):831-839. Christensen B, Mosdol A, Retterstol I, et al. Abstention from filtered coffee reduces the concentration of plasma homocysteine and serum cholesterol-a randomized controlled trial. Am J Clin Nutr 2001;74(3):302-307. Higdon JV, Frei B. Coffee and health: a review of recent human research.Crit Rev Food Sci Nutr. 2006; 46(2):101-123. Hallström H, Wolk A, Glynn A, Michaëlsson K. Coffee, tea and caffeine consumption in relation to osteoporotic fracture risk in a cohort of Swedish women.Osteoporos Int. 2006;17(7):1055-1064.

60. Spiegel K, Leproult R, Van Cauter EV. Impact of sleep debt on metabolic and endocrine function. Lancet 1999;354(9188);1435-1439.

61. Colantuoni C, Rada P, McCarthy J, et al. Evidence that intermittent, excessive sugar intake causes endogenous opioid dependence. Obes Res. 2002;10(6):478-488. Rada P, Avena NM, Hoebel BG. Daily bingeing on sugar repeatedly releases dopamine in the accumbens shell. Neuroscience 2005;134(3):737-744.

62. Link LB, Potter JD. Raw versus cooked vegetables and cancer risk. Cancer Epidemiol Biomarkers Prev. 2004;13(9):1422-1435. Franceschi S, Parpinel M, La Vecchia C, et al. Role of different types of vegetables and fruit in the prevention of cancer of the colon, rectum, and breast. Epidemiology 1998;9(3):338-341. McEligot AJ, Rock CL, Shanks TG, et al. Comparison of serum carotenoid responses between women consuming vegetable juice and women consuming raw or cooked vegetables. Cancer Epidemiol Biomarkers Prev. 1999;8(3):227-231.

63. Key TJA, Thorogood M, Appleby PN, Burr ML. Dietary habits and mortality in 11,000 vegetarians and health conscious people: results of a 17-year follow up. BMJ 1996;313:775-779.

64. Rolls BJ, Roe LS,Meegns JS. Salad and satiety: energy density and portion size of a first-course salad affect energy intake at lunch. J Am Diet Assoc. 2004;104(10):1570-1576.

65. Unlu NZ, Bohn T, Clinton SK, Schwartz SJ. Carotenoid absorption from salad and salsa by humans is enhanced by the addition of avocado or avocado oil. J Nutr. 2005;135(3):431-436.

66. Steinmetz KA, Potter JD. Vegetables, fruit, and cancer prevention: a review. J Am Diet Assoc. 1996;96(10):1027-1039. Genkinger JM, Platz EA, Hoffman SC, et al. Fruit, vegetable, and antioxidant intake and all-cause, cancer, and cardiovascular disease mortality in a community-dwelling population in Washington County, Maryland. Am J Epidemiol. 2004;160(12):1223-1233.

67. Bugianesi R, Salucci M, Leonardi C, et al. Effect of domestic cooking on human bioavailability of naringenin, chlorogenic acid, lycopene and betacarotene in cherry tomatoes. Eur J Nutr. 2004; 43(6):360-366.

68. Halton TL, Willett WC, Liu S, et al. Potato and french fry consumption and risk of type 2 diabetes in women. Am J Clin Nutr. 2006;83(2):284-290.

69. Jansen MC, Bueno-de-Mesquita HB, Feskens EJ, et al. Quantity and variety of fruit and vegetable consumption and cancer risk. Nutr Cancer. 2004;48(2):142-148.

70. Lau FC, Shukitt-Hale B, Joseph JA. The beneficial effects of fruit polyphenols on brain aging. Neurobiol Aging. 2005;26(Suppl 1):128-132.

71. Gorinstein S, Caspi A, Libman I, et al. Red grapefruit positively influences serum triglyceride level in patients suffering from coronary atherosclerosis: studies in vitro and in humans. J Agric Food Chem. 2006;54(5):1887-1892. Aviram M, Rosenblat M, Gaitini D, et al. Pomegranate juice consumption for 3 years by patients with carotid artery stenosis reduces common carotid intima-media thickness, blood pressure and LDL oxidation. Clin Nutr. 2004;23(3):423-433. Duttaroy AK, Jørgensen A. Effects of kiwi fruit consumption on platelet aggregation and plasma lipids in healthy human volunteers. Platelets 2004;15(5):287-292.

72. Blackberry I, Kouris-Blazos A, Wahlqvist ML, et al. "Legumes: the most important dietary predictor of survival in older people of different ethnicities." Asia Pac J Clin Nutr 2004;13(Suppl):S126.

73. Kris-Etherton PM, Hu FB, Ros E, Sabate J. "The role of tree nuts and peanuts in the prevention of coronary heart disease: multiple potential mechanisms." J Nutr 2008;138(9):1746S-1751S.

74. Hu FB, Stampfer MJ. Nut consumption and risk of coronary heart disease: a review of epidemiologic evidence. Curr Atheroscler Rep 1999 Nov;1(3):204-209.

75. Ellsworth JL, Kushi LH, Folsom AR, et al. Frequent nut intake and risk of death from coronary heart disease and all causes in postmenopausal women: the Iowa Women's Health Study. Nutr Metab Cardiovasc Dis. 2001;11(6):372-377. Kris-Etherton PM, Zhao G, Binkoski AE, et al. The effects of nuts on coronary heart disease risk. Nutr Rev. 2001;59(4):103-111.

76. Simopoulos AP. Essential fatty acids in health and chronic disease. Am J Clin Nutr. 1999;70 (3):56S-69S.

77. Rajaram S, Sabat AJ. Nuts, body weight and insulin resistance.Br J Nutr 2006;96 Suppl 2:S79-S86. Sabat ÃJ. Nut consumption and body weight. Am J Clin Nutr 2003;78(3 Suppl):647S-650S. Bes-Rastrollo M, Sabat ÃJ, Gamez-Gracia E, et al. Nut consumption and weight gain in a Mediterranean cohort: The SUN study. Obesity 2007;15(1):107-116. Garc-a-Lorda P, Megias Rangil I, Salas-Salvada J. Nut consumption, body weight and insulin resistance. Eur J Clin Nutr 2003;57 Suppl 1:S8-11. Meg-as-Rangil I, Garc-a-Lorda P, Torres-Moreno M, et al. Nutrient content and health effects of nuts. Arch Latinoam Nutr 2004;54(2 Suppl 1):83-86.

78. Lovejoy JC. The impact of nuts on diabetes and diabetes risk.Curr Diab Rep 2005; 5(5):379-84. Jiang R, Manson JE, Stampfer MJ, Liu S, Willett WC, Hu FB. Nut and peanut butter consumption and risk of type 2 diabetes in women. JAMA 2002; 288(20):2554-2560.

79. Tsai CJ, Leitzmann MF, Hu FB, Willett WC, Giovannucci EL. Frequent nut consumption and decreased risk of cholecystectomy in women. Am J Clin Nutr 2004; 80(1):76-81. Tsai Cj, Leitzmann Me, Hu FB, et al. A prospective cohort study of nut consumption and the risk of gallstone disease in men. Am J Epid 2004;160(10):961-968.

80. Liu S, Sesso HD, Manson JE, et al. Is intake of breakfast cereals related to total and cause-specific mortality in men? Am J Clin Nutr. 2003;77(3):594- 599. Liu S. Intake of refined carbohydrates and whole grain foods in relation to risk of type 2 diabetes mellitus and coronary heart disease. J Am Coll Nutr. 2002;21(4):298-306. Gross LS, Li L, Ford ES, Liu S. Increased consumption of refined carbohydrates and the epidemic of type 2 diabetes in the United States: an ecologic assessment. Am J Clin Nutr. 2004;79(5):774-779. Prentice AM. The emerging epidemic of obesity in developing countries. Int J Epidemiol. 2006;35(1):93-99.

81. Bravi F, Bosetti C, DalMaso L, et al. Macronutrients, fatty acids, cholesterol, and risk of benign prostatic hyperplasia. Urology 2006;67(6):1205-1211.

························ **E** ·······················

High Blood Pressure. *See* **Blood Pressure**

Hormones, 85

Hummus

Black Bean Hummus, 298

Fresh Beet Hummus, 299

Herbed White Bean Hummus, 302

Tasty Hummus, 306

Hunger

Exercise and, 162

Food Addictions and, 81, 146

Four Dimensions of, 115–116

Nutritarian Diet-Style and, 11, 18, 49

Nuts, Seeds and Avocado and, 156

Toxic Hunger, 120–122, 145, 163–164, 178

True Hunger, 122–126, 129

Volume and, 126

Hypertension. *See* **Blood Pressure**

Hypoglycemia, 120, 124

························· **I** ·························

IGF-1, 137, 140, 141, 415, 423

Immune System, 13, 45, 48, 49, 134, 151, 200, 415

Indigestion, 10, 19, 142

Inflexible Palate Syndrome, 99

Insulin, 40, 41, 137, 140, 426. *See also* Diabetes

Irritable Bowel Syndrome, 200

························· **J** ·························

Japan, 52, 136

Juice Recipes

High Cruciferous Juice, 255

Mixed Vegetable Juice, 256

Refreshing Sunrise Juice, 257

························· **K** ·························

Kale

Apple Cinnamon Butternut Squash Soup, 307

Braised Kale and Squash with Pumpkin Seeds, 334

California Creamed Kale, 336

Creamed Forest Kale over Wild Rice, 338

Creamy Cruciferous Curry, 312

Cruciferious Vegetables and, 152

Dr. Fuhrman's Famous Anti-Cancer Soup, 314

Golden Austrian Cauliflower Cream Soup, 317

Great Greens, 346

Green Machine, 347

High Cruciferous Juice, 255

High Cruciferous Vegetable Stew, 318

Kale Pesto over Pasta and Beans, 350

Mediterranean Bean and Kale Sauté, 353

Mixed Vegetable Juice, 256

Nutrient Density Score, 55

Orange Sesame Kale, 357

Pita stuffed with Seasoned Greens, 363

Supreme Kale, 373

Kidney Disease, 25, 182

Mango

Meat. *See* **Animal Foods**

Medication

Menus

Mercury,

Metabolism,

Micronutrients

·················· **O** ··················

························ T ························

························ **W** ························

Walnuts

Watercress

Weight Gain

Weight Loss